American Hospital English (AHE)®

American Hospital English (AHE)®

Picture Book and Pronunciation Guide

Laura Medlin

Copyedited and indexed by D. Lazo

Library of Congress Control Number: 2014900682
ISBN: Hardcover   978-1-4931-6267-3
               Softcover   978-1-4931-6266-6
               eBook   978-1-4931-6268-0

This book was printed in the United States of America.

Rev. date: 04/08/2014

To order additional copies of this book, contact:
Xlibris LLC
1-888-795-4274
www.Xlibris.com
Orders@Xlibris.com
540698

Dedication

to all those who work in the caring professions.

Preface

This book is arranged in alphabetical order. Each of the twenty-six chapters is devoted to one letter of the English alphabet. There are no color examples because this book is printed in black and white. Phonetic spellings have been derived from the International Phonetic Alphabet (IPA). Professional medical illustrations have been obtained from *Old-Time Anatomical Illustrations CD-ROM and Book* (New York, Dover Publications Inc., 2005), edited by Jim Harter. All other illustrations are by the author. This is an introductory and partial list of some of the words, symbols, and images encountered in the American hospital and healthcare environments.

A special thank you to Gail and everyone at FedEx Office for your kindness and expertise!

Introduction

Hello, and welcome to the *American Hospital English (AHE) ® Picture Book and Pronunciation Guide*!

This book is designed for anyone who is interested in the type of language used in American hospitals and healthcare institutions. It contains common everyday language as well as some slang terms and can be useful as a reference tool or exercise book. Many of the sample sentences can be heard in the hospital or in healthcare classes. Remember that everyday speech doesn't always follow perfect grammar rules. The language of healthcare is vast, and this is only an introductory and partial list of words and phrases you may see and hear.

The words, phonetic spellings, definitions, and sample sentences will be in the left-hand margin of each page. Corresponding images and abbreviations will be on the right.

Each entry should contain

    — a phonetic spelling,
    — a definition or explanation, and
    — a sample sentence in quotes that incorporates a form of the words or symbols.

Cover the words and try to identify the pictures. Cover the pictures and practice the words. Practice reading, writing, and speaking the sentences. Make flash cards. Quiz each other. Have fun!

English Alphabet with Phonetic Pronunciations

1. **Aa** \eɪ\	2. **Bb** \bɪ:\	3. **Cc** \sɪ:\	4. **Dd** \dɪ:\	5. **Ee** \ɪ:\
6. **Ff** \ef\	7. **Gg** \dʒɪ:\	8. **Hh** \eɪtʃ\	9. **Ii** \aɪ\	10. **Jj** \dʒeɪ\
11. **Kk** \keɪ\	12. **Ll** \el\	13. **Mm** \em\	14. **Nn** \en\	15. **Oo** \əʊ\
16. **Pp** \pɪ:\	17. **Qq** \kju:\	18. **Rr** \ɑ:\	19. **Ss** \es\	20. **Tt** \tɪ:\
21. **Uu** \ju:\	22. **Vv** \vɪ:\	23. **Ww** \'dʌ-bəl-ju:\	24. **Xx** \eks\	25. **Yy** \waɪ\	26. **Zz** \zɪ:\

There are twenty-six letters in the English alphabet. Each chapter is devoted to one letter. Each chapter has a letter plate as its title.

Pronunciation Key

The phonetic pronunciations provided have been created by and are based solely on the author's interpretation of common English usage in the state of California. The symbols used are derived from those of the International Phonetic Alphabet (IPA). Readers are strongly encouraged to consult with an English-speaking friend or coworker for help with pronunciation.

— **Phonetic spellings** will appear after the word between two slanted lines (\\) like this: **spellings** \'spe-lɪ:ŋz\
— **Syllables** will be separated by a hyphen (-) like this: **syllables** \'sɪl-ə-bəlz\.
— **Accented syllables** will be marked with an apostrophe (') like this: **accented** \'æk-sen-təd\

Vowel Sounds

iː s<u>ee</u>	**ɪ** s<u>i</u>t	**ʊ** f<u>oo</u>t	**uː** f<u>oo</u>d
ɪə <u>ear</u>	**eɪ** x-r<u>ay</u>	**e** t<u>e</u>st	**ə** <u>A</u>meric<u>a</u>
ɜː n<u>ur</u>se	**ɔː** c<u>or</u>ds	**ʊə** fl<u>uoro</u>	**ɔɪ** b<u>oy</u>
əʊ c<u>o</u>lon	**æ** st<u>a</u>t	**ʌ** bl<u>oo</u>d	**ɑː** st<u>ar</u>t
ɒ h<u>o</u>t	**eə** <u>air</u>	**aɪ** cr<u>y</u>o	**aʊ** n<u>ow</u>

Consonant Sounds

tʃ chest	**dʒ** juice	**Θ** thirst	**ð** the
ʃ shock	**ʒ** measure	**ŋ** lung	**ʔ** statin
p pain	**b** bone	**t** tablet	**d** drug
k kidney	**g** glucose	**f** femur	**v** virus
s sodium	**z** plasma	**m** medicine	**n** neuro
h health	**l** liver	**r** renal	**w** water	**j** yawn

Examples: **American** \ə-'meə-ə-kɪn\ **Hospital** \'hɒs-pɪ-dəl\ **English** \'ɪ:ŋ-lɪʃ\
(AHE) \eɪ-eɪʧ-'ɪ:\

Explanation of Symbols and Notes

(*abbrev.*) = **abbreviation** \ə-brɪ:-vɪ:-'eɪ-ʃən\
An **abbreviation** is a shortened version of a word or phrase. Abbreviations are used to save time in talking, listening, reading, and writing. Abbreviations can be initials or symbols.
Example: thyroid-stimulating hormone becomes **TSH** \tɪ:-es-'eɪʧ\ (pronounce each letter)

(*acronym*) = **acronym** \'æ-krə-nɪm\
An **acronym** is a new word formed by the initial letters of each word of a term or phrase.
Example: positive end-expiratory pressure becomes **PEEP** \pɪ:p\ (pronounce as one word)

SYN = **synonym** \'sɪ-nə-nɪm\
A **synonym** is a word that means the same as another.
Example: cranium. **SYN**: skull

ANT = **antonym** \'æn-tə-nɪm\
An **antonym** is a word that means the opposite of another word.
Example: hot. **ANT**: cold.

® = a **registered** trademark or brand name \'re-dʒɪ-stɜ:d\
Example: *Bandaid* ® is a **brand name** for an adhesive bandage.

Latin = a medical term derived from the **Latin language** \'læ-ʔən\ or \'læ-tən\ \'læŋ-wɪdʒ\
Example: **NPO** is from the **Latin** *non per os*, which means "nothing by mouth."

(*n.*) = **noun** \naʊn\
A **noun** is a name for something—a person, place, or thing. Most of the words listed in the following chapters are nouns.
Example: body (*n.*)

(*s.*) = a **singular** form of a noun \'sɪ:ŋ-ju:-lɜ:\
Singular means just one thing.
Example: one foot (*s.*)

(*pl.*) = the **plural** form of a noun \'plɜ:-əl\
Plural means more than one thing.
Example: two feet (*pl.*)

(*adj.*) = the **adjective** or descriptive form of a word \'æ-dʒek-tɪv\
Example: abdomen (*n.*) abdominal (*adj.*)

Recommended Books

The following are all excellent books on the subjects of English language, medicine, and healthcare, particularly in the United States. Please use these books to look up further information on any words presented here:

1. *The Oxford Picture Dictionary (Monolingual English)*
   author: Shapiro and Adelson-Goldstein
   publisher: Oxford University Press

2. *Merriam-Webster's Collegiate Dictionary*, eleventh edition
   author: Merriam-Webster
   publisher: Merriam-Webster

3. *Taber's Cyclopedic Medical Dictionary*, twenty-first edition
   author: Donald Venes
   publisher: F. A. Davis Company

4. *Harrison's Principles of Internal Medicine*, eighteenth edition
   author: Long, Fauci, Kasper, Hauser, Jameson, and Loscalzo
   publisher: McGraw-Hill

5. *Medical Terminology: A Short Course*, sixth edition
   author: Davi-Ellen Chabner
   publisher: Saunders

6. *Anatomy and Physiology*, seventh edition
   author: Patton and Thibodeau
   publisher: Mosby

Chapter One

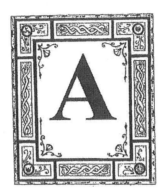

Aa \eɪ\
The letter *A* is the first letter of the English alphabet.

A is for *apple* \'æ-pəl\.
"An **apple** a day keeps the doctor away."

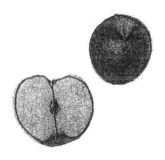

ABD
\eɪ-biː-ʼdiː\ a thick, absorbent wound
dressing
"An **ABD** pad is often used on surgical
incisions."

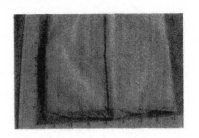

abdomen
\ʼæb-də-mən\ the region of the body
between the thorax and the pelvis that
holds the stomach, liver, intestines,
kidneys, gallbladder, and spleen SYN:
belly, stomach.
"Assessment of the **abdomen** includes
palpation."

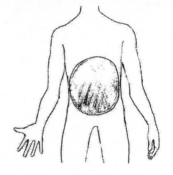

abdominal (*abbrev.*)
\æb-ʼdɒ-mən-əl\ of or pertaining to the
abdomen
"Change **abd**. drsg. QD."

abd.

abdominal aortic aneurysm (*abbrev.*)
\trɪ-pəl- ʼeɪ\ an abnormal dilation of a
section of the aorta
"**AAA** repair is a major surgery."

AAA.

abduction
\æb-ʼdʌk-ʃən\ the moving of a limb
away from the center of the body
"The opposite of **abduction** is
adduction."

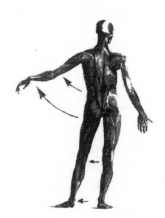

above
\ə-'bʌv\ in or to a higher place
"There's a light switch **above** the bed."

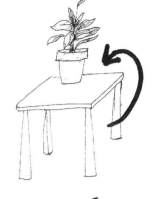

above-the-knee amputation
\ə-'bʌv ɵə nɪ: æmp-ju:-'teɪ-ʃən\ the
removal of a leg above the knee joint by
surgery or trauma
"He had an **above-the-knee amputation**
after an MVA."

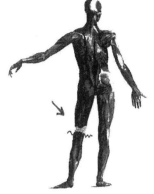

above-the-knee amputation (*abbrev.*)
\eɪ-keɪ-'eɪ\
"An **AKA** patient will have a wrapped
thigh stump."

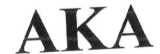

acetabulum
\æ-sɪ-'tæb-ju:-ləm\ a concave socket on
the side of the hip bone
"The head of the femur sits inside the
acetabulum to form the hip joint."
acetabular (*adj.*).

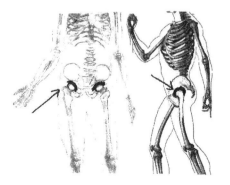

acetylsalicylic acid (*abbrev.*)
\eɪ-es-'eɪ\ a chemical compound that
reduces fever and relieves pain SYN:
aspirin.
"Ingesting too much **ASA** can cause GI
bleeding."

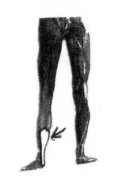

ASA

Achilles tendon
\ə-'kɪ-lɪːz 'ten-dən\ a large tendon
that connects the calf muscles
(gastrocnemius and soleus) to the heel
bone (calcaneus)
"The patient cannot walk due to a
ruptured **Achilles tendon.**"

acid-fast bacilli (*abbrev.*)
\eɪ-ef-'bɪː\ a certain type of bacteria and
its staining properties
"An **AFB** smear is one test for TB."
bacillus (*s.*)

AFB

acquired immunodeficiency syndrome
(*acronym*)
\eɪdz\ complications arising from
infection with HIV
"An **AIDS** patient is very susceptible to
opportunistic infections."

AIDS

acromion process
\ə-'krəʊ-mɪː-ən 'prɒ-ses\ a point of the
shoulder blade (scapula) that articulates
with the humerus to form the shoulder
"The **acromion process** is one landmark
for an IM injection in the deltoid
muscle."

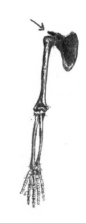

activities of daily living (*abbrev.*)
\eɪ-dɪ:-'elz\
"**ADLs** include eating, bathing, and getting dressed."

ADL's

acute coronary syndrome (*abbrev.*)
\eɪ-sɪ:-'es\ any group of symptoms arising from blocked coronary arteries
"The patient complaining of chest pain was admitted with a diagnosis of **ACS**."

ACS

acute lymphocytic leukemia (*abbrev.*)
\eɪ-el-'el\ a cancer of the white blood cells
"A patient with **ALL** will have an elevated WBC count."

ALL

acute myeloid leukemia (*abbrev.*)
\eɪ-em-'el\ a type of bone marrow cancer
"The patient with **AML** was placed in protective isolation."

AML

acute myocardial infarction (*abbrev.*)
\ə-'kju:t em-'ɑɪ\ a current heart attack
"The patient was admitted with a diagnosis of **AMI**."

AMI

acute renal failure (*abbrev.*)
\eɪ-ɑ:-'ef\ a disorder of the kidneys
"Severe dehydration can cause **ARF**."

ARF

acute tubular necrosis (*abbrev.*)
\eɪ-tɪ:-'en\ a condition of renal failure
"Severe dehydration can cause **ATN**."

ATN

Adam's apple
\'æ-dəmz 'æ-pəl\ a bump on the front of
the neck formed by the thyroid cartilage
of the larynx SYN: larynx, voice box.
"Men generally have a larger **Adam's
apple** than women."

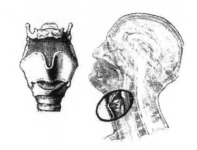

adduction
\'æ-dʌk-ʃən\ the moving of a limb
toward the center of the body
"**Adduction** is the opposite of
abduction."

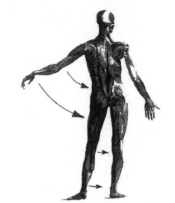

adhesive bandage
\æd-'hi:-sɪv 'bæn-dɪdʒ\ a small gauze
dressing with tape attached
"A commonly used brand name for an
adhesive bandage is *Bandaid* ®
\'bæn-deɪd\."

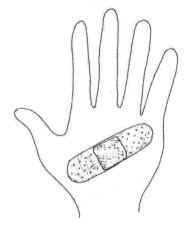

adipose tissue
\'æ-dɪ-pəʊz 'tɪ-ʃu:\ fat
"Liposuction is a procedure that
removes **adipose tissue**."

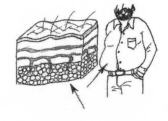

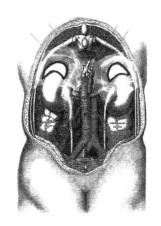

adrenal glands
\ə-'drɪ:-nəl glænz\ two glands that sit
on top of the kidneys
"Catecholamines are produced by the
adrenal glands."

adult respiratory distress syndrome
(*acronym*)
\ɑ:dz\ a disorder of breathing
"Peritonitis can lead to **ARDS**."

ARDS

advanced cardiac life support
(*abbrev*.)
\eɪ-sɪ:-el-'es\ a group of emergency
medical procedures performed in the
event of cardiopulmonary arrest
"**ACLS** certification is required every
two years."

ACLS

aerosol mask
\'eə-ə-sɒl mæsk\ a plastic device that
delivers moist air
"Asthma patients may benefit from an
aerosol mask."

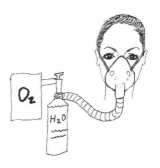

**against medical advice or American
Medical Association** (*abbrev*.)
\eɪ-em-'eɪ\
"The patient chose to leave the hospital
AMA."
"That doctor is a member of the **AMA**."

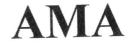

airway
\'eə-weɪ\ the passageway for air to enter and exit the lungs SYN: trachea.
"It's important to maintain a patent **airway** in a sedated patient."

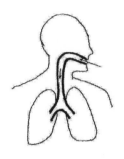

alanine aminotransferase (*abbrev.*)
\eɪ-el-'tɪ:\ an enzyme in the blood
"An elevated **ALT** level may indicate liver disease."

ALT

alpha
\'æl-fə\ the first letter of the Greek alphabet.
"Some **alpha**-blockers can be used to lower blood pressure."

α

alveoli
\æl-'vɪ:-əʊ-lɑɪ\ air sacs of the lungs
"Smoking can damage the **alveoli**."
alveolus (*s.*), **alveolar** (*adj.*).

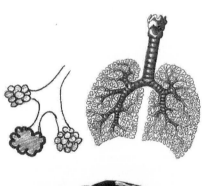

Ambu bag
\'æm-bu:-bæg\ a handheld device that delivers positive pressure ventilations SYN: bag valve mask (BVM).
"Keep an **Ambu bag** in every patient room."

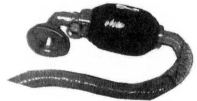

ambulance
\'æm-bju:-ləns\ a vehicle to transport sick or injured people to the hospital
"Another name for an **ambulance** is EMS."

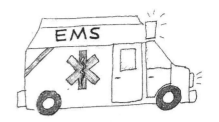

ambulate
\'æm-bju:-leɪt\ walk
"The patient can **ambulate** with physical therapy."
ambulatory (*adj.*).

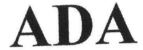

American Diabetes Association
(*abbrev.*)
\eɪ-dɪ:-'eɪ\
"An **ADA** diet may also be called a *consistent carbohydrate diet.*"

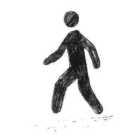

the symbol for **ammonia**
\ə-'məʊn-jə\ a substance formed by the breakdown of nitrogen-containing proteins and amino acids
"Liver failure may cause an elevated serum NH_3 level."

amniotic fluid
\æm-nɪ:-'ɒ-dɪk 'flu:-ɪd\ the clear fluid that surrounds a fetus during pregnancy.
"Rupturing of membranes and release of **amniotic fluid** is called *water breaking.*"

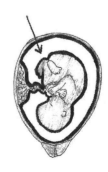

ampule
\'æmp-ju:l\ a small glass vial that holds
medications for injection
"Meds in a glass **ampule** should be
drawn up with a filter needle."

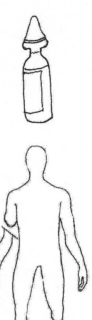

amputation
\æmp-ju:-'teɪ-ʃən\ the removal of a limb
or body part by surgery or trauma.
"The patient's foot had to be **amputated**
due to gangrene."

amyotrophic lateral sclerosis (*abbrev.*)
\eɪ-el-'es\ a motor-neuron disease that
causes weakness and muscle atrophy
"**ALS** is also called *Lou Gehrig's
disease*."

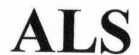

aneurysm
\'æn-jɜ:-ɪ-zəm\ an abnormally dilated
area of a blood vessel
"The patient died from a ruptured
cerebral **aneurysm**."

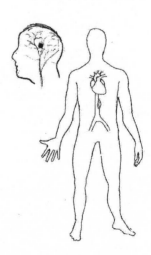

angioplasty
\ˈæn-ʤɪ:-əʊ-plæs-tɪ:\ a procedure that opens narrow or blocked blood vessels
"The patient had an **angioplasty** with stent placement."

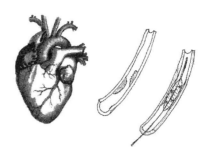

angiotensin-converting enzyme inhibitor (*abbrev.*)
\eɪs-ɪn-ˈhɪ-bɪ-dɜ:\ a class of blood pressure medications
"The patient is allergic to **ACEI**."

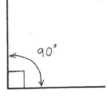

angle
\ˈæŋ-əl\ a figure formed by two lines extending from the same point or corner
"Ninety degrees is a right **angle**."

angry
\ˈæŋ-rɪ:\ the emotions of anger; mad
"The patient is **angry** because he can't have salt in his food."

anion gap (*abbrev.*)
\ˈæn-ɑɪ-ən gæp\ a calculation used in assessing metabolic acidosis.
"An **AG** is monitored in DKA."

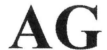

ankle
\ˈæn-kəl\ the joint between the leg and the foot SYN: tarsus.
"The patient will need crutches due to a broken **ankle**."

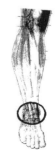

ante cibum
\eɪ-ˈsɪː\ Latin for "before meals."
"The patient has blood sugar checks
ordered **ac** & HS."

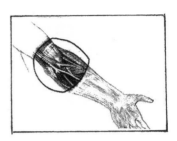

antecubital fossa
\æn-tə-ˈkjuː-bɪ-dəl ˈfɒs-ə\ the area of
the arm at the inner elbow
"Blood is often drawn from veins in the
antecubital fossa region."
fossae (*pl.*)

ante meridiem
\ˈeɪ-em\ Latin for morning; the time
period from midnight to 12:00 noon.
"Take one tablet daily in **a.m.**"

anterior
\æn-ˈtɪə-ɪ:-ɜ:\ the front of the body.
"**Anterior** is the opposite of *posterior*."

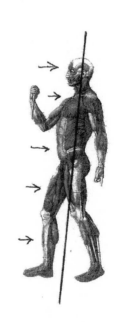

anterior cruciate ligament (*abbrev.*)
\eɪ-sɪː-ˈel\ tissue that connects the thigh
bone (femur) to the lower leg bone
(tibia) inside the knee
"Many athletes have **ACL** injuries."

anterior-posterior (*abbrev.*)
\eɪ-'pɪ:\ from front to back
"An **AP** chest x-ray is a single view."

AP

antibiotic-resistant microorganisms
(*abbrev.*)
\eɪ-ɑ:-'em\ a name for certain types of
microorganisms, such as MRSA
"The patient is in contact isolation for
ARM."

ARM

antidiuretic hormone (*abbrev.*)
\eɪ-dɪ:-'eɪʧ\ a pituitary hormone that
acts on the kidneys
"Another name for **ADH** is
vasopressin."

ADH

antinuclear antibody (*abbrev.*)
\eɪ-en-'eɪ\
"An **ANA** level may be ordered to help
diagnose autoimmune disorders."
antibodies (*pl.*)

ANA

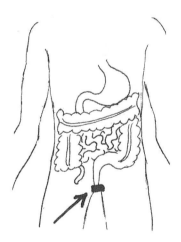

anus
\'eɪ-nəs\ the outlet of the rectum that
lies between the buttocks
"Care should be taken in neutropenic
patients to keep the **anal** area clean."
anal (*adj.*)

aorta
\eɪ-'ɔ:-də\ the main artery of the body
originating from the left ventricle
"The **aorta** is the largest artery in the
body."

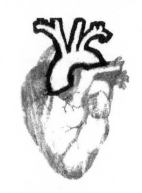

aortic valve
\eɪ-'ɔ:-dɪk væElv\ the heart valve
between the left ventricle and the aorta
"Aortic stenosis is a disease of the
aortic valve."

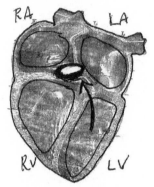

appendix
\ʌ-'pen-dɪks\ a worm-shaped piece of
the intestine at the end of the cecum
"Inflammation of the **appendix** is called
appendicitis."

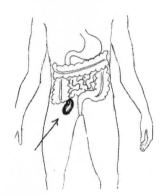

applesauce
\'æ-pəl-sɒs\ a food item made of
cooked and pureed apple
"The patient swallows pills with
applesauce."

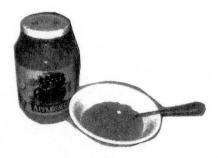

April (*abbrev.*)
\'eɪ-prəl\ the fourth month of the year
"**Apr.** showers bring May flowers."

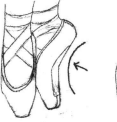

arch
\aːʧ\ the curved inner aspect of
the bottom of the foot. Also called
longitudinal arch
"Some foot pain may be relieved by the
use of **arch** supports."

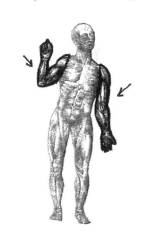

arm
\aːm\ the upper extremity from the
shoulder to the hand.
"Blood pressure is usually measured on
the upper **arm**."

armpit
\'aːm-pɪt\ the area under the shoulder
between the arm and the thorax
SYN: axilla, underarm.
"The **armpit** has sweat and scent
glands."

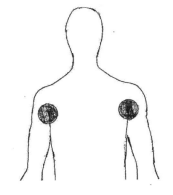

arrow
\'eə-əʊ\ a symbol to indicate direction.
"Street signs use **arrows** to direct the
flow of traffic."
arrows (*pl.*)

arterial blood gas (*abbrev.*)
\eɪ-biː-'dʒiː\ a blood test.
"An **ABG** checks the pH of the body."

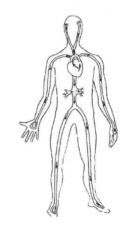

artery
\'ɑː-dɜː-ɪː\ any of the vessels that carry
blood from the heart to the tissues
"An **artery** is usually deeper than a
vein."
arteries (*pl.*)

ascites
\ə-'sɑɪ-diːz\ the abnormal collection of
fluid in the peritoneal cavity
"One symptom of liver cirrhosis is
ascites."

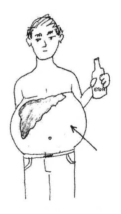

aspartate aminotransferase (*abbrev.*)
\eɪ-es-'tiː\ an enzyme involved in amino
acid and carbohydrate metabolism
"An elevated **AST** level may indicate
liver disease."

aspirate
\'æs-pɜ:-eɪt\ to inhale fluid or food into the lungs
"CVA patients may **aspirate** thin liquids."

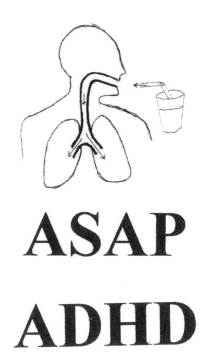

as soon as possible (*abbrev.*)
\eɪ-es-eɪ-'pɪ:\ SYN: STAT.
"Please bring the supplies **ASAP**."

ASAP

attention-deficit hyperactivity disorder (*abbrev.*)
\eɪ-dɪ:-eɪtʃ-'dɪ:\
"Many children are diagnosed with **ADHD**."

ADHD

atrial fibrillation (*abbrev.*)
\'eɪ-trɪ:-əl fɪ-brɪ-'leɪ-ʃən\ an abnormal heart rhythm marked by irregular electrical activity and quivering of the atria
"The patient was admitted with rapid **AF**."

AF

atelectasis
\æ-də-'lek-tə-sɪs\ a collapsed or airless condition of the lung
"**Atelectasis** is a potential complication of bedrest after surgery."

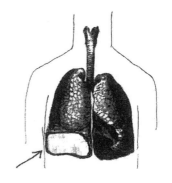

atherosclerosis
\æ-ɵɜ:-əʊ-sklɜ:-'əʊ-sɪs\ a condition
of plaque deposits in the walls of the
arteries
"A high lipid concentration in the blood
can lead to **atherosclerosis**."

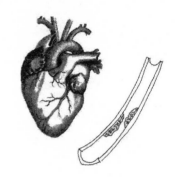

atrial fibrillation
\'eɪ-trɪ:-əl fɪ-brɪ-'leɪ-ʃən\ a cardiac
rhythm marked by irregular electrical
activity and quivering of the atria SYN:
AF.
"The patient is anticoagulated due to
atrial fibrillation."

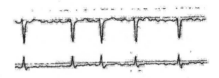

atrioventricular block (*abbrev.*)
\eɪ-vɪ:-'blɒk\ a condition of the
electrical conduction of the heart
"First degree **AVB** is defined by a P-R
interval greater than 0.20 sec on an EKG
strip."

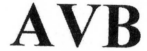

AVB

atrium
\'eɪ-trɪ:-əm\ one of two top chambers
of the heart "There is a blood clot in the
right **atrium**."
atria (*pl.*), **atrial** (*adj.*)

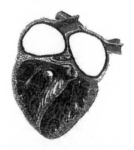

August (*abbrev.*)
\'ɒ-gəst\ the eighth month of the year
"**Aug.** is a summer month."

Aug.

auricle
\'ɔ:-ɪ-kəl\ the outer ear
"The patient has several piercings in the left **auricle**."

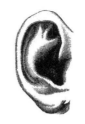

auscultation
\ɒ-skəl-'teɪ-ʃən\ listening for sounds within the body
"**Auscultation** is one part of a physical examination."

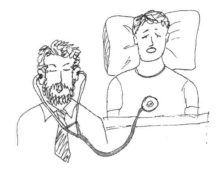

automated external defibrillator
\eɪ-ɪ:-'dɪ:\ a portable device that analyzes heart rhythms and delivers electric shocks
"Most shopping malls have an **AED** on site."

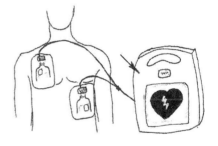

automated external defibrillator
(*abbrev.*)
\eɪ-ɪ:-'dɪ:\ a portable device that analyzes heart rhythms and delivers electric shocks
"Turn on the **AED** and follow the instructions."

AED

automated implanted cardiac defibrillator (*abbrev.*)
\eɪ-ɑɪ-sɪ:-'dɪ:\ an implanted device that delivers electric shocks
"The patient has an **AICD** and a pacemaker."

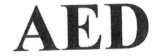

AICD

axillary (*abbrev.*)
\'æk-səl-eə-ɪ:\ of or relating to the area
under the arm
"Take an **axillary** temp if the patient has
had something cold to drink."

axilla
\æk-'sɪl-ə\ the region under the shoulder
between the arm and the ribcage
SYN: armpit, underarm.
"Put an ice pack in the **axilla** to help
bring his fever down."
axillae (*pl.*), **axillary** (*adj.*)

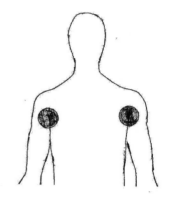

Chapter Two

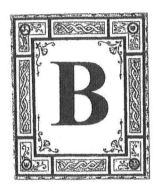

Bb \bɪː\
The letter *B* is the second letter of the English alphabet.

B is for *baby*. \'beɪ-bɪː\
"Don't throw the **baby** out with the bath water."

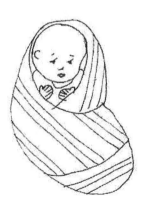

belladonna and opium (*abbrev.*)
\bɪ:-en-'əʊ\ medications
"A **B&O** suppository may help relieve
bladder pain."

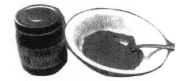

baby bottle
\'beɪ-bɪ: 'bɒ-dəl\ a container for a baby
to drink from
"Disposable **baby bottles** are used in
the hospital."
bottles (*pl.*)

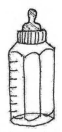

baby food
\'beɪ-bɪ: fu:d\ food suitable for a baby
to eat
"*Pureed* is the consistency of **baby
food**."

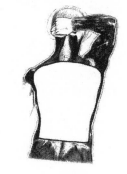

back
\bæk\ posterior part of the upper body;
dorsum
"**Back** is the opposite of *front*."

backbone
\'bæk-bəʊn\ the vertebral column;
spinal column SYN: spine.
"Check for pressure sores along the
backbone."

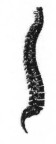

backpack
\'bæk-pæk\ a bag that may be worn on
the back to carry items
"Many young people carry **backpacks**."
backpacks (*pl.*)

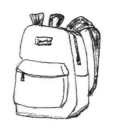

bag valve mask (*abbrev.*)
\bæg vælv 'mæsk\ a piece of
respiratory equipment
SYN: Ambu bag.
"Use of a **BVM** is part of ACLS
instruction."

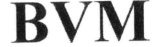

bald
\bɒld\ hairless
"Many young men are **bald** these days
because they shave their heads."

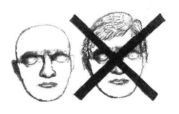

balloon
\bə-'lu:n\ a flexible, expandable object
"The urinary catheter has a **balloon** on
the end."

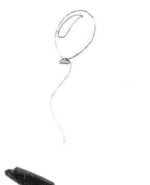

ballpoint pen
\'bɒl-pɔɪnt pen\ a writing implement
with a metal tip and ink
"A **ballpoint pen** is used to write on
medical documents."

banana
\bə-'næ-nə\ a type of yellow tropical fruit
"**Bananas** are rich in potassium."
bananas (*pl.*)

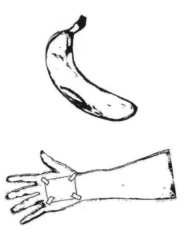

bandage
\'bæn-dɪʤ\ a piece of fabric used to cover and bind up wounds
"Another word for **bandage** is *dressing*."

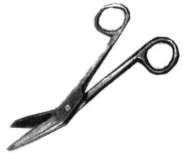

bandage scissors
\'bæn-dɪʤ 'sɪ-zɜːz\ scissors with a rounded tip for cutting close to the skin
"**Bandage scissors** are safest to use with patients."

the symbol for the element **barium**
\'beə-ɪ:-əm\ refer to the periodic table of the elements
"A **barium** enema takes a picture of the large intestine."

Ba++

basic life support (*abbrev.*)
\bɪ:-el-'es\ resuscitative measures
"The patient was transported to another facility with **BLS** protocol."

BLS

basic metabolic panel (*abbrev.*)
\bɪ:-em-'pɪ:\ a blood chemistry test
"Get a **BMP** to check the patient's electrolytes."

BMP

basilic vein
\bə-'sɪ-lɪk veɪn\ the large vein on the
inner side of the biceps
"The **basilic vein** is one vein used for
an IV site."

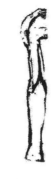

basin
\'beɪ-sən\ a plasic container to hold
water for washing
"The patient's toiletries are kept inside
their wash **basin**."

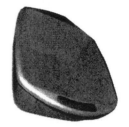

bassinet
\bæ-sɪ-'net\ a small bed for a baby
"Newborn infants are kept in a
bassinet."

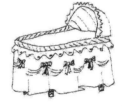

battery
\'bæ-dʒ-rɪ:\ a single cell that produces
electric current
"Hearing aid **batteries** need to be
replaced regularly."
batteries (*pl.*)

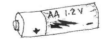

beard
\brəd\ facial hair that grows on the chin
and cheeks
"A BiPAP mask may not seal properly if
the patient has a **beard**."

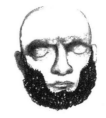

bed
\bed\ a piece of furniture to lie and sleep on
"We have three **beds** available for new admits."
beds (*pl.*)

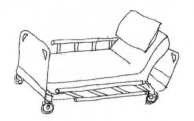

bedpan
\'bed-pæn\ a receptacle for urine and feces
"A **bedpan** is used when the patient is on bedrest."

bedside commode (*abbrev.*)
\'bed-sɑɪd kʌ-'məʊd\ a portable toilet
SYN: commode, potty chair.
"Bedrest with **BSC**."

BSC

bedside commode
\'bed-sɑɪd kə-'məʊd\ a portable toilet
SYN: potty chair, BSC.
"The patient has been getting up on the **bedside commode**."

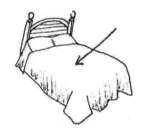

bedspread
\'bed-spred\ a decorative cloth cover for a bed
"The patient requested the **bedspread** be removed because he was too warm."

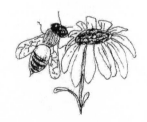

bee
\biː\ an insect that produces honey and beeswax
"**Bees** make honey."
bees (*pl.*)

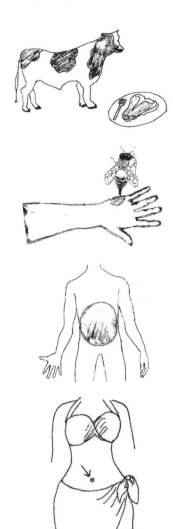

beef
\bɪːf\ the meat of the cow
"**Beef** is considered red meat."

bee sting
\'bɪː stɪːŋ\ an injury caused by the
stinger of a bee
"Some patients are allergic to **bee
stings**."
stings (*pl.*)

belly
\'be-lɪː\ abdomen SYN: stomach.
"The patient is complaining of **belly**
pain."

belly button
\'be-lɪː bʌ-ʔən\ the abdominal scar from
the umbilical cord
SYN: umbilicus, navel.
"Many young women have **belly button**
piercings nowadays."

below
\bə-'ləʊ\ underneath an object or
surface
"Cups are kept in the cupboard **below**
the ice machine."

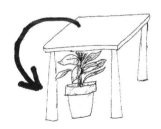

below-the-knee amputation
\bɪ:-keɪ-'eɪ\ the severing of a leg below
the knee joint by surgery or trauma
"The abbreviation for **below-the knee amputation** is BKA."

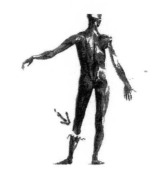

belt
\belt\ a piece of flexible material worn
around the waist
"I need to wear a **belt** now that I've lost
weight."

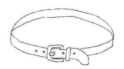

bend
\bend\ to turn or force from straight or
even to curved or angular SYN: flex.
"The opposite of **bend** is *straighten*."

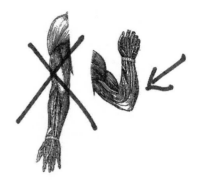

benzodiazepines (*abbrev.*)
\'ben-zəʊz\ a class of sedative
medications.
"*Diazepam* and *lorazepam* are two
kinds of **benzos**."

benzos

beta
\'beɪ-də\ the second letter of the Greek
alphabet
"Metoprolol is a **beta**-adrenergic
blocker."

β

beveled
\'be-vəld\ a surface cut with a slanted
edge
"Large needles are usually inserted
beveled side down."

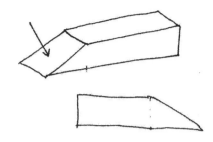

the formula for **bicarbonate**
\bɑɪ-'kɑ:-bə-neɪt\ a buffering agent in
the body
"Start an IV gtt with **HCO$_3$**."

HCO3-

biceps
\'bɑɪ-seps\ the muscle of the upper arm
that flexes the elbow and supinates the
forearm
"Bodybuilders like to flex their **biceps**."

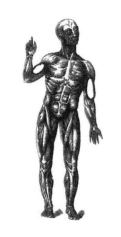

bicuspid valve
\bɑɪ-'kʌs-pɪd vælv\ heart valve
between the left atrium and left ventricle
SYN: mitral valve.
"The **bicuspid valve** has two leaflets."

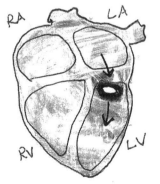

bicycle
\'baɪ-sɪ-kəl\ a vehicle with two wheels and pedals to propel it
"A shorter name for **bicycle** and motorcycle is *bike*."

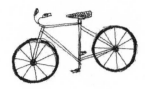

bifurcation
\baɪ-fɜ:-'keɪ-ʃən\ division into two branches
"Insert the needle above that **bifurcation**."

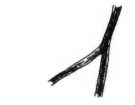

bigeminy
\baɪ-'dʒem-ə-nɪ:\ occurring in pairs or couplets
"In ventricular **bigeminy**, every other beat is a PVC."

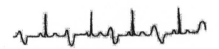

big toe
\bɪg 'təʊ\ the first toe of the foot. SYN: hallux, great toe.
"I stubbed my **big toe**."

biohazard
\baɪ-əʊ-'hæ-zɜ:d\ anything that is harmful or potentially harmful to humans, other species, or the environment
"Blood and body fluids go in the **biohazard** trash."

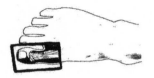

biopsy (*abbrev.*)
\'baɪ-ɒp-sɪ:\ a surgical procedure to test tissue
"The doctor needs supplies for a needle **bx**."

Bx

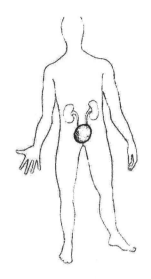

bladder
\'blæ-dɜ:\ the reservoir for urine in the body
"The patient has a distended **bladder**."

blanket
\'blæn-kət\ a large piece of woven fabric used to cover a bed or the body
"The patient is cold and requests a warm **blanket**."

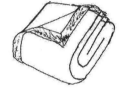

bleach
\blɪːʧ\ a liquid preparation of chlorine
"**Bleach** is a disinfectant."

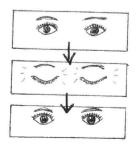

blink
\blɪːnk\ involuntary shutting and opening of the eye
"A normal response to a corneal stimulation test is a **blink**."

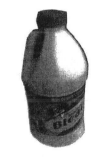

blood clot
\'blʌd klɒt\ a coagulated mass of blood
"Keep the SCDs on to prevent a **blood clot**."

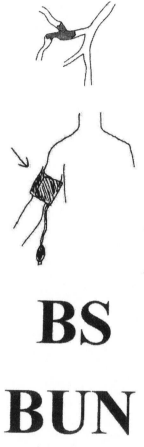

blood pressure cuff
\blʌd 'pre-ʃɜ: kʌf\ an inflatable device
used to measure blood pressure
SYN: BP cuff.
"The patient doesn't want the **blood pressure cuff** on the same side where she had her mastectomy."

blood sugar; bowel sounds (*abbrev.*)
\blʌd 'ʃʊ-gɜ:\ \'baʊ-əl saʊnz\ serum
glucose; intestinal activity
"Active **BS** heard in all four quadrants."

BS

blood urea nitrogen (*abbrev.*)
\bɪ:-ju:-'en\ a blood chemistry test
"**BUN** is one measurement of renal function."

BUN

bowel movement (*abbrev.*)
\bɪ:-'em\ defecation
"When was the patient's last **BM**?"

BM

bobby pins
\'bɑ-bɪ: pɪnz\ flat wire hairpins with
prongs that press close together
"**Bobby pins** should be removed while a patient is sleeping to prevent injury."

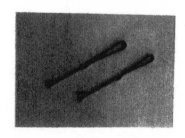

body mass index (*abbrev.*)
\bɪ:-em-'aɪ\ a weight calculation
"**BMI** is one measure of obesity."

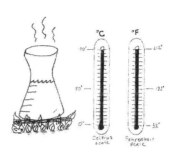

boiling
\'bɔɪ-lɪ:ŋ\ heated to the boiling point
212 F or 100 C.
"**Boiling** is the opposite of *freezing*."

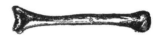

bone
\bəʊn\ dense, connective osseous tissue
"The word root for **bone** is *osteo*."

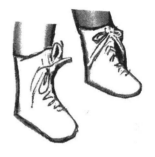

boots
\bu:ts\ apparel for the feet usually
reaching above the ankle
"He died with his **boots** on."

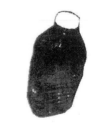

bottle
\'bɒ-dəl\ a container for liquids
"Can I have a squirt **bottle** for washing
please?"

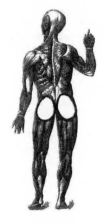

bottom
\'bɒ-dəm\ buttocks
"Scoot your **bottom** over a little more
this way."

bow
\bəʊ\ a decorative knot
"That's a pretty **bow** you have in your
hair."

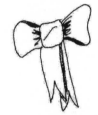

bowel
\'baʊ-əl\ the intestines SYN: gut.
"The absence of **bowel** sounds is an
abnormal finding."

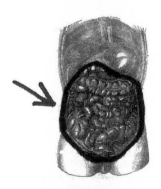

bowl
\bəʊl\ a basin-shaped dish for food
"All I want is a **bowl** of soup."

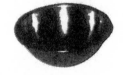

box

\bɒks\ a rigid, typically rectangular container

"They're kept in that **box** on the top shelf."

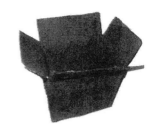

blood pressure (*abbrev.*)

\bɪ:-'pɪ:\ a hemodynamic measurement

"Pain can cause an elevated **BP**."

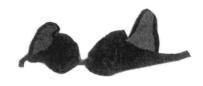

bra

\brɒ\ an undergarment for women worn on the upper torso

"The patient would like to keep her **bra** on."

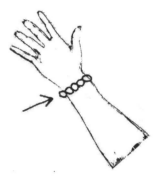

bracelet

\'breɪs-lət\ a piece of jewelry worn on the wrist

"The patient's **bracelet** was placed in the hospital safe."

brachial

\'breɪ-kɪ:-əl\ pertaining to the arm

"A **brachial** site pulse is checked on infants."

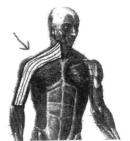

braids
\breɪdz\ hair that has three or more
strands interwoven
"Would you like your hair done with
two **braids** while you are in bed?"

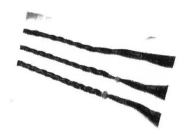

brain
\breɪn\ a large soft mass of nerve tissue
contained within the cranium
SYN: cerebrum.
"The word root for **brain** is *neuro*."

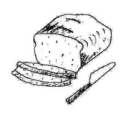

bread
\bred\ a usually baked and leavened
food made with flour
"A patient with celiac disease cannot
tolerate the gluten in many types of
bread."

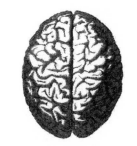

brainstem
\'breɪn-stem\ the stemlike part of
the brain that connects the cerebral
hemispheres with the spinal cord
"The comatose patient was determined
to only have **brainstem** function."

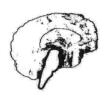

brainstem auditory evoked response
(abbrev.)
\beə\ a diagnostic test of brain activity
"A **BAER** may be ordered for CVA
patients."

BAER

break
\breɪk\ fracture
"Another use of the word *break* is to
indicate a rest period for workers."
broken (*adj.*)

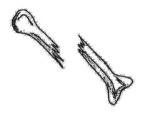

breast
\brest\ mammary gland
"The patient is complaining of **breast**
tenderness."

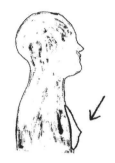

breastbone
\'brest baʊn\ sternum
"I banged my **breastbone** into the
steering wheel in the accident."

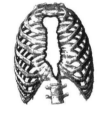

breastfeeding
\'brest-fɪ:-dɪːŋ\ the giving of mother's
milk to an infant
"**Breastfeeding** is the best nutrition for
newborns."

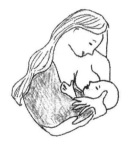

brick
\brɪk\ a rectangular-shaped block used
in building or paving
"The patient sustained head injuries
when his car crashed into a **brick** wall."

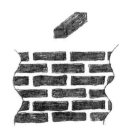

briefs

\brɪːfs\ men's underpants
"Boxer shorts and **briefs** are two types
of men's underwear."

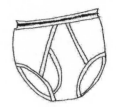

bronchials

\'brɒn-kɪː-əlz\ the airways from the
trachea into the lungs
"This medicine will help open up your
bronchials."

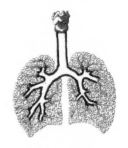

broom

\bruːm\ a bundle of firm, stiff fibers
bound together on a long handle for
sweeping
"The floor was swept with a **broom**."

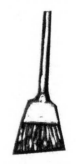

bruise

\bruːz\ an injury that ruptures small
blood vessels without breaking the skin
"Patients on blood thinners can **bruise**
easily."

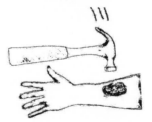

brush

\brʌʃ\ a utensil with bristles for
smoothing the hair SYN: hairbrush.
"I should have a **brush** in that bag."

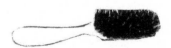

bucket

\'bʌ-kət\ a typically cylindrical
container for catching, holding, or
carrying liquids or solids
"A mop and **bucket** are used to clean
the floor."

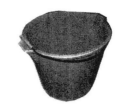

Buck's traction

\bʌks 'træk-ʃən\ extension of a wrapped
limb with weights
"**Buck's traction** may reduce spasms
from a hip fracture."

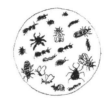

bugs

\bʌgz\ insects or microbes
"This foam will help kill any **bugs** on
your hands."

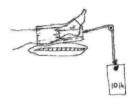

bulb drain

\bʌlb dreɪn\ a tube that removes fluid
from a part of the body SYN: JP.
"A **bulb drain** applies gentle suction to
a surgical site."

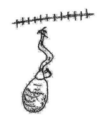

bulb syringe

\bʌlb sə-'rɪndʒ\ a rounded device that
removes fluids from a body cavity by
applying suction
"A **bulb syringe** is used to clear nasal
secretions from an infant."

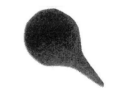

bullet

\'bʌl-ət\ the ammunition for a gun
"The **bullet** has lodged in his brain."

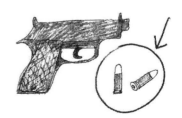

bundle branch block
\'bʌn-dəl bræntʃ blɒk\ a defect in the
heart's electrical conduction with a QRS
complex measuring longer than 0.12 sec
SYN: BBB.
"The patient is in sinus rhythm with a
bundle branch block."

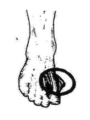

bundle branch block (*abbrev.*)
\'bʌn-dəl bræntʃ blɒk\ one aspect of
electrical conduction in the heart
"A **BBB** is defined as a QRS longer
than 0.12 sec."

BBB

bunion
\'bʌn-jən\ inflammation and thickening
of the first metatarsal joint of the big toe
"I have **bunions** from always wearing
high heels."
bunions (*pl.*)

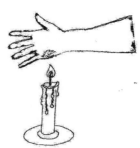

burn
\b3:n\ tissue injury caused by exposure
to heat, fire, or chemicals
"**Burns** can easily get infected and must
be cared for properly."
burns (*pl.*)

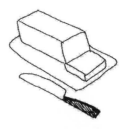

butter
\'bʌ-dɜ:\ the fatty product of churned
milk or cream
"**Butter** is made from milk fat."

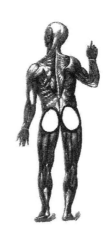

buttocks

\'bʌ-dəks\ the fleshy areas posterior to
the hips SYN: bottom.
"There is one pressure sore on the left
buttocks."

button

\'bʌ-ʔən\ usually a circular fastener for
clothing
"**Buttons** are a choking hazard for
infants and children."
buttons (*pl.*)

Chapter Three

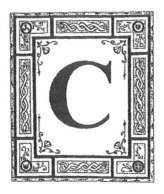

Cc \sɪ:\
The letter *C* is the third letter of the English alphabet.

C is for *cat*. \kæt\
"Curiosity killed the **cat**."

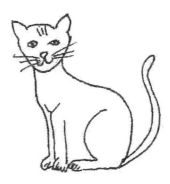

caduceus
\kæ-'duː-səs\ a generic symbol of medicine
"That medical snake symbol thing is called a *caduceus*."

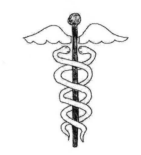

caffeine, alcohol, pepper, aspirin-free
(*acronym*)
\'kæ-pə frɪː\ a diet order
"A **CAPA-free** diet is ordered to help decrease stomach irritation."

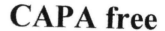

cake
\keɪk\ a sweet baked food made from dough or thick batter
"**Cake** and ice cream are traditional American birthday foods."

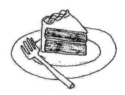

calcaneus
\kæl-'keɪ-nɪː-əs\ the heel bone
"The patient's left **calcaneus** was crushed in the MVA."

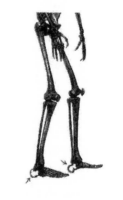

the formula for **calcium chloride**
\'kæl-sɪː-əm 'klɔː-ɑɪd\ a chemical given to raise serum calcium
"Give him one amp of **CaCl** please."

the symbol for the **calcium** ion
\'kæl-sɪ:-əm\ a chemical in the body
"Check a serum **Ca++** please."

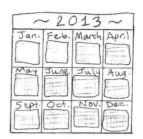

calendar
\'kæl-en-dɜ:\ an orderly list of days and
months
"Let me check the **calendar** to see if
I'm working that day."

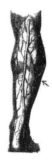

calf
\kæf\ the posterior portion of the leg
below the knee
"The patient is complaining of cramping
in his **calves**."
calves (*pl.*)

call bell
\kɒl bel\ a signaling device to elicit help
in the hospital SYN: call light.
"I'll put your **call bell** right here in your
lap."

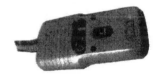

call light
\kɒl lɑɪt\ a signaling device to elicit
help in the hospital SYN: call bell.
"Your **call light** is on. Do you need
something?"

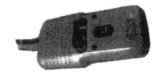

camera
\'kæm-rə\ a device that takes
photographs
"A **camera** is used to document a
patient's wounds."

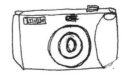

cancer (*abbrev.*)
\'kæn-sɜ:\ a condition of malignant
cells in the body
"The patient has a history of prostate
CA."

CA

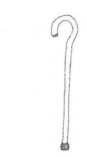

cane
\keɪn\ a walking stick
"The patient is unsteady on his feet and
walks with a **cane**."

capnogram
\'kæp-nəʊ-græm\ an ETCO2
waveform
"A capnogram is monitored during
anesthesia."
capnography (*n.*), SYN

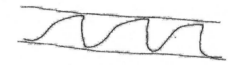

capsule
\'kæp-su:l\ a container made of gelatin
for a single dose of a drug
"Lactobacillus usually comes in **capsule**
form."

carbohydrates (*abbrev.*)
\kɑ:-bəʊ-'haɪ-dreɪts\ foods that are a
source of energy
"Diabetic patients need to keep track of
their **CHO** consumption."

CHO

the symbol for the element **carbon**
\'kɑ:-bən\ refer to the periodic table of
the elements
"The formula for *carbon monoxide* is
CO."

C

the formula for **carbon dioxide**
\sɪ:-əʊ-'tu:\ an acid in the body
"**CO$_2$** is a waste product of
metabolism."

CO2

carcinoembryonic antigen (*abbrev.*)
\sɪ:-ɪ:-'eɪ\ a serology test
"**CEA** is one cancer marker."

CEA

cardiac output (*abbrev.*)
\'kɑ:-dɪ:-æk 'aʊt-pʊt\ a measure of
heart function
"Decreased **C.O.** may cause poor renal
perfusion."

C.O.

cardiopulmonary resuscitation
(*abbrev.*)
\sɪ:-pɪ:-'ɑ:\ a set of life-saving
interventions
"**CPR** certification is required every
two years."

CPR

carotid
\kə-'rɒ-dəd\ an artery on either side of
the neck that supplies blood to the head
"A **carotid** pulse is checked during
CPR."

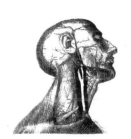

carpus
\'kɑ:-pəs\ the eight bones of the wrist
joint SYN: wrist.
"Many people have **carpal** tunnel
surgery to help with hand discomfort."
carpal (*adj.*)

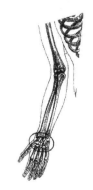

cart
\kɑ:t\ a small wheeled vehicle
"The lunch trays are on the **cart**."

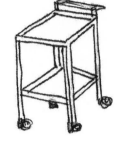

cast
\kæst\ a usually plaster mold applied to
a body part to immobilize a broken bone
"All his friends have signed his **cast**."

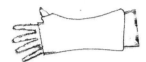

cataract
\'kæ-dɜ:-ækt\ an opacity of the lens of
the eye
"I've had **cataract** surgery done on both
eyes."

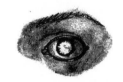

catheter
\'kæ-ɵɘ-dɜ:\ a tube that drains urine
from the bladder
"A commonly used brand name for a
catheter is *Foley®*."

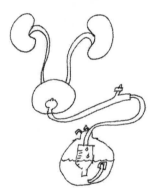

cath tip syringe
\kæɵ tɪp sɘ-'rɪnʤ\ a large syringe with
a long smooth tip for flushing
"A **cath tip syringe** is used to flush an
NG tube."

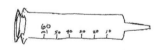

cecum
\'sɪ:-kəm\ a pouch that forms the first part of the large intestine
"The appendix attaches to the **cecum**."

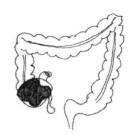

cell phone
\'sel fəʊn\ a small portable telephone
"Most people today carry **cell phones**."
phones (*pl.*)

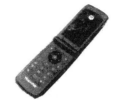

centimeter (*abbrev.*)
\'sen-ə-mɪ:-dʒ:\ a metric unit of length
"A six-foot-tall man is 183 **cm** in length."

central venous pressure (*abbrev.*)
\sɪ:-vɪ:-'pɪ:\ a hemodynamic measure
"**CVP** monitoring can help determine fluid status."

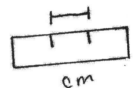

cerebral aneurysm
\sə-'rɪ:-brəl 'æn-jɜ:-ɪ-zəm\ an abnormal dilation of a blood vessel inside the brain
"Uncontrolled hypertension is one risk factor for developing a **cerebral aneurysm**."

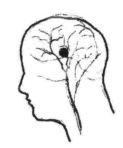

central nervous system (*abbrev.*)
\sɪ:-ən-'es\ the brain and spinal cord
"Caffeine is a **CNS** stimulant."

cerebral palsy; chest pain (*abbrev.*)
\sɪ:-'pɪ:\ symptoms of a brain injury;
angina
"Give NTG 0.4 mg SL prn **CP**."

CP

cerebral perfusion pressure (*abbrev.*)
\sɪ:-pɪ:-'pɪ:\ a measure of blood flow to
the brain
"It is important to maintain adequate
CPP in stroke patients."

CPP

cerebellum
\seə-ə-'bel-əm\ the largest section of
the hindbrain
"The **cerebellum** plays a role in
coordination and balance."

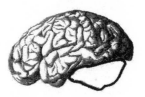

cerebrospinal fluid (*abbrev.*)
\sɪ:-es-'ef\ the fluid that surrounds the
brain and spinal cord
"**CSF** needs to be analyzed on
meningitis patients."

CSF

cerebrum
\sə-'rɪ:-brəm\ the largest portion of the
brain SYN: brain.
"There are two **cerebral** hemispheres—
left and right."
cerebral (*adj.*)

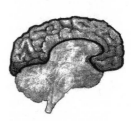

certified nurse assistant (*abbrev.*)
\sɪ:-en-'eɪ\ title
"The **CNA** will hand out meal trays."

CNA

cervical collar
\'sɜ:-vɪ-kəl 'kɒ-lɜ:\ a device used to
immobilize or support the neck
"C-spine precautions include the use of
a **cervical collar**."

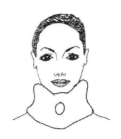

cervical spine
\'sɜ:-vɪ-kəl spɑɪn\ the bones of the neck
SYN: neck.
"**Cervical spine** injuries can cause
paralysis."

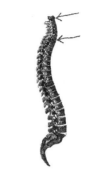

cervix
\'sɜ:-vɪks\ the neck and lower portion of
the uterus
"**Cervix** dilation is monitored during
labor."

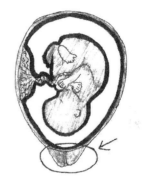

chair
\tʃeə\ a seat with four legs and a back
designed for one person
"Would you like to sit in the **chair** for
breakfast?"

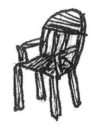

change
\ˈʧeɪnʤ\ coins; money left over from a transaction
"I have some **change** in my pocket."

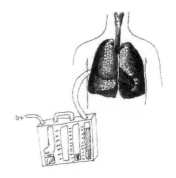

chart
\ˈʧɑːt\ a collection of patient information
"Do you have the patient's **chart**?"

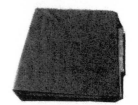

cheek
\ʧɪːk\ the side of the face below the eye
"Your **cheeks** are flushed."
cheeks (*pl.*)

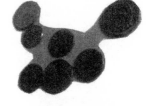

chest of drawers
\ˈʧest-ə-drɔːz\ an upright piece of furniture with drawers for storing clothes
SYN: dresser
"Please put my purse in that **chest of drawers**."

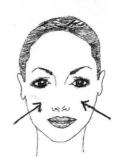

chest tube
\ˈʧest tuːb\ a drain placed in the pleural space to drain air or fluid
"A **chest tube** is placed after lobectomy surgery to collect drainage."

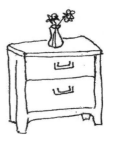

chest-tube clamp
\ʧest tuːb klæmp\ a device used to cut
off the flow of a chest tube
"Keep a **chest-tube clamp** at the
bedside of a patient who has a chest
tube."

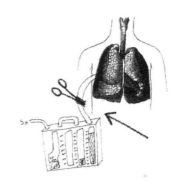

chest
\ʧest\ the thorax
"I'm feeling heaviness in my **chest**."

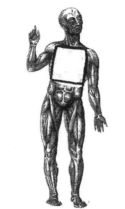

chest x-ray (*abbrev.*)
\ʧest 'eks-reɪ\ a radiologic image of the
chest
"Get a STAT portable **CXR**."

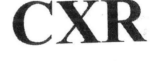

chewing gum
\'ʧuː-ɪːŋ gʌm\ a sweetened and flavored
material designed for chewing
SYN: gum.
"I don't want you to fall asleep with
chewing gum in your mouth because
you might choke."

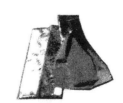

chicken
\'ʧɪ-kən\ the common domestic fowl
"**Chicken** is also called *poultry*."

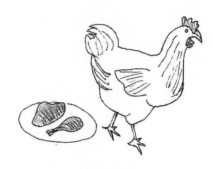

chin
\ʧɪn\ the point of the lower jaw
"A cleft in the **chin**, the devil within."

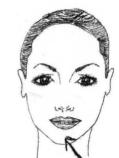

the symbol for the **chloride** ion
\'klɔ:-ɑɪd\ an electrolyte in the body
"**Cl⁻** is an electrolyte found in body
fluids."

chronic kidney disease (*abbrev.*)
\sɪ-keɪ-'dɪ:\ a condition of renal
impairment
"The patient with **CKD** may also be
anemic."

chronic lymphocytic leukemia
(*abbrev.*)
\sɪ:-el-'el\ a bone marrow disease
"**CLL** is a disease of the bone marrow."

chronic myelogenous leukemia
(*abbrev.*)
\sɪ-em-'el\ a bone marrow disease
"**CML** is a cancer of the white blood
cells."

Cl-

CKD

CLL

CML

chronic obstructive pulmonary disease (*abbrev.*)
\sɪ:-əʊ-pɪ:-'dɪ:\ a lung disease
"**COPD** can cause chronic CO_2 retention."

COPD

chronic renal failure (*abbrev.*)
\sɪ:-ɑ:-'ef\ a condition of renal impairment
"She has **CRF** and has just started getting dialysis."

CRF

cigarettes
\'sɪ-gə-rets\ a slender roll of cut tobacco inside paper to be smoked
"Smoking **cigarettes** can cause lung damage."

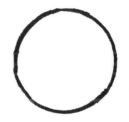

circle
\'sɜ:-kəl\ a round ring shape
"The *circle of Willis* is an arterial structure in the brain."

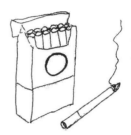

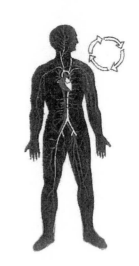

circulation
\sɜ:-kju:-'leɪ-ʃən\ the movement of
blood through the vessels of the body
"Capillary refill is one way to check
circulation."

circumflex artery (*abbrev.*)
\'sɜ:-kəm-fleks\ one of the coronary
arteries
"There is an occlusion in the mid
CMX."

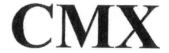

clavicle
\'klæ-vɪ-kəl\ the bone that connects
with the sternum and the scapula
SYN: collar bone.
"The subclavian vein lies below the
clavicle."

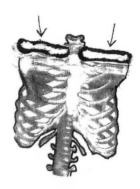

clipboard
\'klɪp-bɔ:d\ a small writing board with a
clip at the top for holding papers
"I need a **clipboard** for this consent."

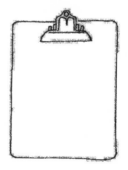

clock
\klɑk\ a device that indicates or measures time
"There's a **clock** on that wall."

clothes
\kləʊz\ garments that are worn
"His **clothes** are in the closet."

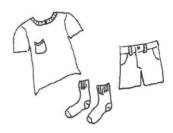

coat
\kəʊt\ an outer garment for keeping warm
"Put your **coat** on because it's cold outside."

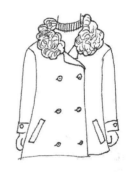

coccyx
\'kɒk-sɪks\ the small bone at the base of the spinal column SYN: tailbone.
"She has a stage I pressure sore on her **coccyx**."

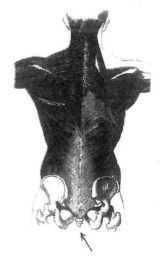

cochlea
\'kəʊ-klɪː-ə\ a portion of the middle ear
"His deafness is caused by damage to
the **cochlea**."
cochlear (*adj.*)

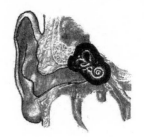

coffee
\'kɒ-fɪː\ a beverage made from the
roasted and ground seeds of the coffee
plant
"Let's make a fresh pot of **coffee**."

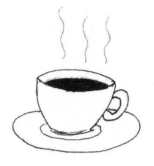

coil
\kɔɪl\ a series of loops; spiral
"The NG tube was **coiled** inside the
esophagus."
coiled (*adj.*)

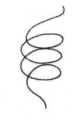

coins
\kɔɪnz\ round metal money SYN:
change.
"I only have **coins**, no paper money
with me."

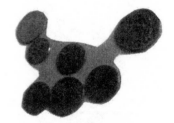

cold
\kəʊld\ a condition of low temperature
"**Cold** is the opposite of hot."

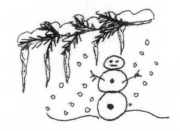

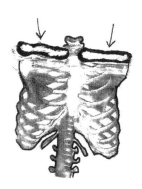

collarbone
\'kɒ-lɜ: bəʊn\ the bone that connects
with the sternum and the scapula
SYN: clavicle.
"He crashed his bike and broke his
collarbone."

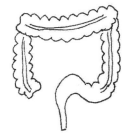

colon
\'kəʊ-lən\ the large intestine
"The patient has a hx of **colon** CA."

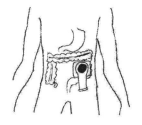

colostomy
\kə-'lɒ-stə-mɪ:\ a surgical opening
in a portion of the colon through the
abdominal wall
"The **colostomy** is draining well."

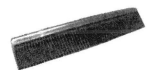

comb
\kəʊm\ a utensil for smoothing the hair
"Let's **comb** your hair."

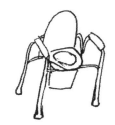

commode
\kə-'məʊd\ a receptacle suitable for use
as a toilet SYN: BSC, potty chair.
"She gets up on the **commode** to void."

complete blood count (*abbrev.*)
\sɪ:-bɪ:-'sɪ:\ a hematology test
"Get a **CBC** after the blood transfusion is completed."

CBC

computed tomography (*abbrev.*)
\sɪ:-'tɪ:\ a radiologic image
"A head **CT** was done to rule out cerebral bleeding."

CT

computer information systems (*abbrev.*)
\sɪ:-ɑɪ-'es\ the computer engineering department
"I had to call **CIS** because my computer froze up."

CIS

computerized provider order entry (*abbrev.*)
\sɪ:-pɪ:-əʊ-'ɪ:\ a system of medical data entry
"The doctors place orders via **CPOE**."

CPOE

computer on wheels (*acronym*)
\kɑʊ\ a portable computer
"The nurses use the **COW**s to deliver meds to each patient."

COW

concave
\'kɒn-keɪv\ curving inward
"The opposite of **concave** is *convex*."

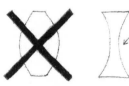

cone
\kəʊn\ a shape or solid with a circular base and a narrow, pointed top
"Put out the orange rubber **cones** when the floor is wet."
cones (*pl.*) **conical** (*adj.*)

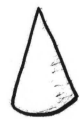

congestive heart failure (*abbrev.*)
\sɪ:-eɪʧ-'ef\ a heart condition
"**CHF** symptoms include shortness of
breath."

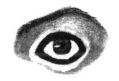

conjunctiva
\kʌn-'ʤʌnk-tə-və\ the mucous
membrane that lines the eyelids
"Some people call red **conjunctiva**
pinkeye."
conjunctival (*adj.*)

continuous (*abbrev.*)
\kən-'tɪn-ju:-əs\ ongoing
"Connect the chest-tube drain to **cont.**
suction."

constriction
\kən-'strɪk-ʃən\ narrowing of a vessel or
opening
"Bright light should cause pupil
constriction."

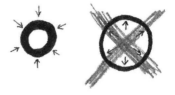

continuous positive air pressure
(*acronym*)
\'sɪ:-pæp\ a respiratory aid
"He wears a **CPAP** at home for sleep
apnea."

contracture
\kʌn-'træk-ʃɜ:\ fibrosis of connective
tissue that prevents normal mobility
"His right arm is **contractured** due to
an old left CVA."
contractured (*adj.*)

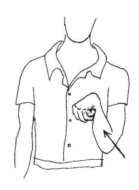

convex

\'kɒn-veks\ curved or rounded outward
"The opposite of **convex** is *concave*."

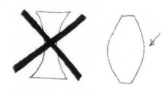

cookies

\'kʊ-kɪːz\ small flat or slightly raised
cakes
"**Cookies** are a popular snack food in
the United States."

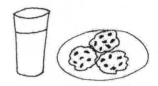

cornea

\'kɔː-nɪː-ə\ the transparent part of the
eyeball that covers the pupil and iris
"Some vision problems can be corrected
by changing the shape of the **cornea**
with a laser."
corneal (*adj.*)

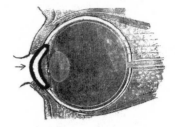

coronary arteries

\'kɔː-ə-neə-ɪː 'ɑː-də-rɪːz\ arteries that
supply blood to the heart muscle
"Angina is one symptom of blocked
coronary arteries."

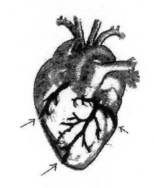

coronary artery bypass graft

\'kɔː-ə-neə-ɪː 'ɑː-dɜː-ɪː 'baɪ-pæs
græft\ surgical establishment of a shunt
that permits blood to flow around a
blocked coronary artery SYN: CABG
"The patient has a history of a **coronary
artery bypass graft** on 4 vessels
(CABG x 4)."

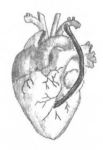

coronary artery bypass graft
(*acronym*)
\'kæ-bɪʤ\ surgery to create a shunt
to bypass blocked arteries and allow
adequate blood flow to the heart
"The patient will need a **CABG** for an
occluded LAD."

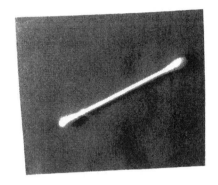

cotton-tipped applicator
\'kɒ-ʔən-tɪpt 'æp-lɪ-keɪ-dɜː\ cotton or
gauze at the end of a slender
stick SYN: swab.
"A commonly used brand name for
cotton-tipped applicator is *Q-tip®*
\kju:-tɪp\."

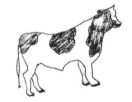

cow
\kaʊ\ a domestic bovine animal
"The **cow** says *moo*."

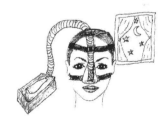

CPAP mask
\'sɪ:-pæp mæsk\ a device (continuous
positive air pressure) worn to alleviate
sleep apnea symptoms
"I brought my own **CPAP** machine
from home."

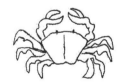

crab
\kræb\ a marine crustacean with pincers
on the front limbs
"**Crab** is one type of shellfish."

crackers
\'kræ-kɜ:z\ a crispy, dry thin baked
bread product
"Graham **crackers** are often served as a
snack in the hospital."

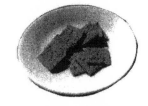

cranium
\'kreɪ-nɪ:-əm\ the portion of the skull
that encloses the brain SYN: skull.
"Infants have an opening in their
cranium called a *fontanel*."
cranial (*adj.*)

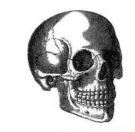

crash cart
\'kræʃ kɑ:t\ a moveable chest that stores
medicines, supplies, and equipment for
life-threatening emergencies
"Unplug the **crash cart** before you
move it."

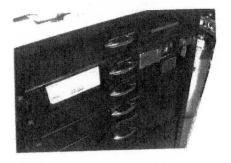

creatine phosphokinase (*abbrev.*)
\sɪ:-pɪ:-'keɪ\ a serology test
"A rhabdomyolysis patient will have an
elevated **CPK**."

CPK

C-reactive protein (*abbrev.*)
\sɪ:-ɑ:-'pɪ:\ a serology test
"An elevated **CRP** may indicate
inflammation."

CRP

crib
\krɪb\ a bed for a baby or small child
"Keep the rails up when the baby is in
the **crib**."

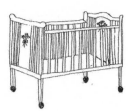

cross
\krɒs\ a figure or mark formed by two intersecting lines crossing at their midpoints
"The American Red **Cross** is a humanitarian organization."

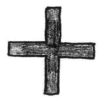

crotch
\krɒʧ\ the area of the groin where the thighs part SYN: groin.
"There is a rash in the **crotch** area."

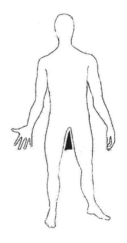

crutches
\'krʌ-ʧəz\ a pair of supports that assist with walking or standing
"The patient will need **crutches** due to a broken ankle."
crutch (*s.*)

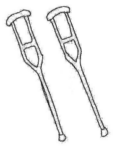

cube
\kju:b\ a shape or solid with six equal square sides
"Oral polio vaccines used to be given with a sugar **cube**."

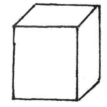

cubic centimeter (*abbrev.*)
\\'kju:-bɪk 'sen-ə-mɪ:-dʒ:\\ or
\\sɪ:-'sɪ:\\ a metric unit of volume
"1 **cc** = 1 ml."

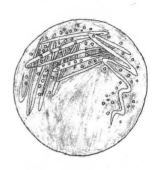

culture
\\'kʌl-ʧɜ:\\ the growing of
microorganisms or living tissue cells in
special media
"Pneumonia patients will have a sputum
gram stain and **culture** done."

culture and sensitivity (*abbrev.*)
\\sɪ:-ən-'es\\ a microbiological test
"Get a UA and a urine **C&S** please."

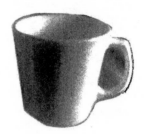

cup
\\kʌp\\ an open bowl-shaped drinking
container
"One **cup** equals eight ounces."

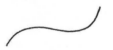

curved
\\kɜ:vd\\ deviating from a straight line
with a smooth turn
"He prefers a **curved** blade for
intubation."

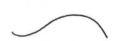

cut

\kʌt\ to penetrate with an edged instrument SYN: laceration.
"A paper **cut** can be an entry site for bacteria on the hands of healthcare workers."

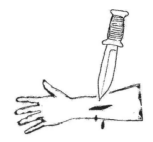

cuticles

\'kju:-dɪ-kəl\ the layer of tissue covering the base of the fingernails
"Healthcare workers should keep their **cuticles** healthy to prevent infection."

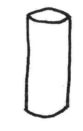

cylinder

\'sɪ-lɪn-dɜ:\ a circular or tubelike shape or solid with two flat ends
"A pill bottle is **cylindrical** in shape."
cylindrical (*adj.*)

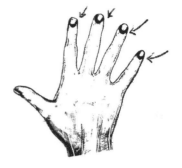

cytomegalovirus (*abbrev.*)

\sɪ:-em-'vɪ:\ a type of virus
"**CMV** is a type of herpes virus."

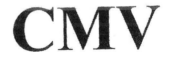

Chapter Four

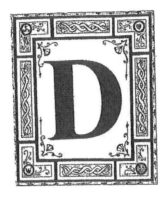

Dd \dɪː\
The letter *D* is the fourth letter of the English alphabet.

D is for *dog*. \dɒg\
"Let sleeping **dogs** lie."

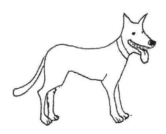

date of birth (*abbrev.*)
\deɪd-ʌv-'bɜ:θ\ the specific month, day, and year of birth
"A nameband will have the patient's **DOB**."

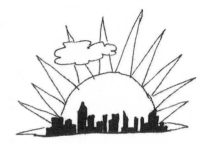

daytime
\'deɪ-tɑɪm\ when the sun is up, from dawn until dusk
"I only drink coffee during the **daytime**."

December (*abbrev.*)
\də-'sem-bɜ:\ the twelfth month of the year
"**Dec.** 25 is Christmas Day."

decerebrate
\dɪ-'seə-ə-brət\ the rigid body position of a patient who has lost cerebral control of spinal reflexes
"With **decerebrate** posturing the arms are extended."

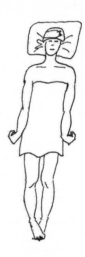

deciliter (*abbrev.*)
\'de-sə-lɪ:-dɜ:\ a metric unit of volume
"Blood sugar is measured in mg/**dl**."

decimal point
\'des-məl pɔɪnt\ a period or centered dot
"Put a zero in front of the **decimal point**."

$$0.0625 \text{ mg}$$

decorticate
\dɪ-'kɔː-də-kət\ the stiff posture of a patient with a lesion at or above the upper brainstem
"With **decorticate** posturing, the arms are flexed."

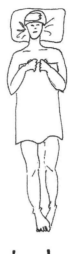

the symbol for **decrease**
\dɪ-'krɪːs\ to lower or reduce in size
"The opposite of **decrease** is *increase*."

deep vein thrombosis (*abbrev.*)
\dɪː-vɪː-'tɪː\ a dangerous blood clot
"Immobility can cause a **DVT**."

DVT

defibrillator
\də-'fɪb-rɪ-leɪ-dʒː\ an electrical device that allows defibrillation of the heart
"A **defibrillator** is kept on every unit."

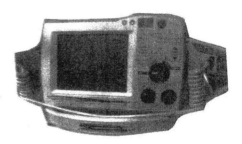

degenerative joint disease (*abbrev.*)
\dɪ:-dʒeɪ-'dɪ:\ a bone disease
"Arthritis is an example of **DJD**."

DJD

delirium tremens (*abbrev.*)
\dɪ:-'tɪ:z\ a group of symptoms related
to alcohol or drug withdrawal
"**DTs** can cause hallucinations and
sweating."

DT's

delta
\'del-tə\ the fourth letter of the Greek
alphabet
"The **delta** symbol is shorthand to
indicate *change*."

deltoid
\'del-tɔɪd\ the large triangular muscle
that covers the shoulder joint
"IM shots can be given in the **deltoid**
muscle."

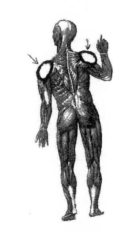

dentition
\den-'tɪ-ʃən\ teeth
"The patient has dental caries and poor
dentition."

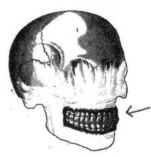

denture cleaner
\'den-ʧɜ: 'klɪ:-nɜ:\ a substance, usually
in tablet form, that cleans and disinfects
dentures
"A commonly used brand name for
denture cleaner is *Efferdent®*
\'e-fɜ:-dent\."

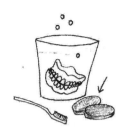

denture cup
\'den-ʧɜ: kʌp\ a container to store or
clean dentures in
"A **denture cup** should be labeled with
the patient's name."

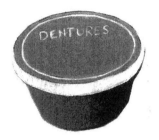

dentures
\'den-ʧɜ:z\ artificial teeth
"**Dentures** are also called *false teeth*."

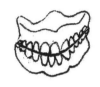

dermatomes
\'dɜ:-mə-təʊmz\ a band or region of
skin supplied by a single spinal nerve
"Shingles usually erupts along one
dermatome."
dermatome (*s.*)

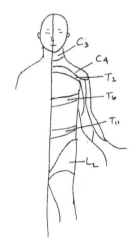

dextrose in water, 50% (*abbrev.*)
\dɪ:-'frf-tɪ:\ a type of sugar
"Intravenous **D50** is given for
hypoglycemia."

D50

dextrose in water, 5% (*abbrev.*)
\dɪ:-fɑɪv-'dʌ-bəl-ju:\ a type of sugar
"Many IV medications are mixed in
D5W."

D5W

dextrose in water, 10% (*abbrev.*)
\dɪ:-'ten\ a type of sugar
"Run some **D10W** until you get the new
TPN bag."

D10W

diabetic ketoacidosis (*abbrev.*)
\dɪ:-keɪ-'eɪ\ a metabolic abnormality
"Urine ketones are monitored in **DKA**."

DKA

diabetes mellitus (*abbrev.*)
\dɑɪ-ə-'bɪ:-dɪ:z 'me-lə-dəs\ a metabolic
disorder marked by hyperglycemia
"One symptom of **DM** is polyuria."

DM

diagonal
\dɑɪ-'æ-gə-nəl\ inclined obliquely from
a reference line; slanted SYN: oblique.
"That confused patient is always lying
diagonally across the bed."
(*diagonally* is an adverb form of the
word)

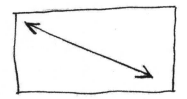

diagnosis-related group (*abbrev.*)
\dɪ:-ɑ:-'dʒɪ:\ a health-care classification
system
"The **DRG** system is a method of
managing the cost of healthcare
services."

DRG

diameter
\dɑɪ-'æ-mə-dɜ:\ the width of a circle
"The inner lumen size of a tube is its
diameter."

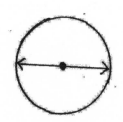

diaper
\'daɪ-pɜ:\ a garment for infants to contain waste matter
"Weigh the baby's **diaper** to measure I&O."

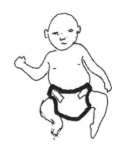

diaphragm
\'daɪ-ə-fræm\ the dome-shaped skeletal muscle that separates the abdomen from the thoracic cavity
"Hiccups are **diaphragm** spasms."

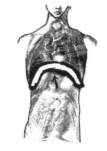

diastolic blood pressure (*abbrev.*)
\daɪ-ə-'stɒ-lɪk blʌd 'pre-ʃɜ:\ the bottom number of a blood pressure measurement
"Keep the **DBP** under 90."

DBP

dicrotic notch
\daɪ-'krɒ-dɪk nɒtʃ\ in a pulse tracing, the notch on the descending limb
"Find the **dicrotic notch** when measuring on the strip."

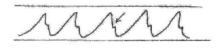

digestive tract
\daɪ-'dʒes-tɪv træk\ the alimentary canal, from the mouth to the colon
"The **digestive tract** may also be called the *intestinal tract*."

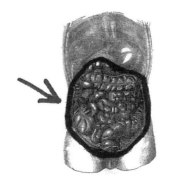

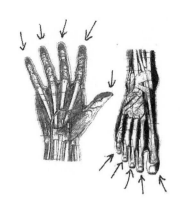

digits
\'dɪ-dʒətz\ fingers and toes
"The adjective referring to any of the
digits is *digital*."

dilation
\daɪ-'leɪ-ʃən\ expansion of an orifice,
organ, or vessel.
"The opposite of **dilation** is
constriction."

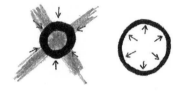

dilation and curettage (*abbrev.*)
\dɪ:-ən-'sɪ:\ a gynecological surgical
procedure
"She had a **D&C** done for excessive
bleeding."

D & C

diphtheria, pertussis, tetanus
(*abbrev.*)
\dɪ:-pɪ:-'tɪ:\ vaccines
"A **DPT** vaccine is standard for children
in the United States."

DPT

disk
\dɪsk\ a flat, round, platelike structure
"A **diskectomy** can relieve chronic neck
or back pain."

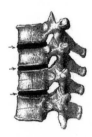

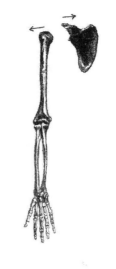

dislocation
\dɪs-ləʊ-'keɪ-ʃən\ the displacement of
any part, especially of a bone, from its
normal position in a joint
"**Dislocation** is the opposite of
articulation."

**disseminated intravascular
coagulation** (*abbrev.*)
\dɪ:-ɑɪ-'sɪ:\ a disorder of blood clotting
"A **DIC** panel includes fibrinogen and
FSP levels."

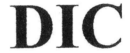

distal
\'dɪs-təl\ farthest from the center
"**Distal** is the opposite of *proximal*."

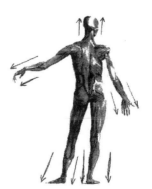

diverticula
\dɑɪ-vɜ:-'tɪk-ju:-lə\ sacs or pouches in
the walls of the colon
"An inflammation of the **diverticula** is
called *diverticulitis*."
diverticulum (*s.*)

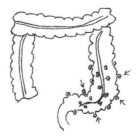

dollar sign
\'dɒ-lɜ: sɑɪn\ a mark placed before a number to indicate that it stands for dollars
"Several **dollar signs** written together usually means that something is expensive."
signs (*pl.*)

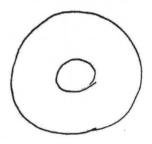

do not resuscitate (*abbrev.*)
\dɪ:-en-'ɑ:\ a life-saving measure/ decision
"The patient has a **DNR** order."

doughnut
\'dəʊ-nʌt\ a small ring shape with a hole in the center; a cake with the same shape
"A **doughnut** seat cushion can help relieve coccyx pain."

down
\daʊn\ toward or in a lower physical position
"**Down** is the opposite of *up*."

drain
\dreɪn\ a tube to drain off fluid or waste products
"A **drain** was placed at the surgical site."

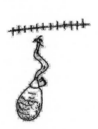

dresser

\'dre-sɜ:\ an upright piece of furniture with drawers for storing clothes SYN: chest of drawers.
"When a small **dresser** is next to the bed, it may be called a *nightstand*."

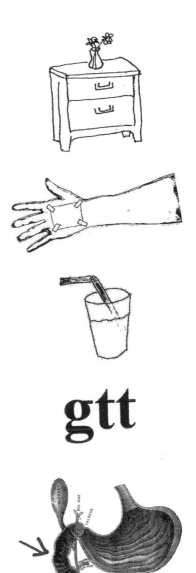

dressing

\'dre-sɪ:ŋ\ a protective covering for injured or diseased parts SYN: bandage.
"The **dressing** is clean, dry, and intact."

drink

\drɪ:nk\ to swallow, or a liquid suitable for swallowing; beverage
"Tuck your chin down when you take a **drink** please."

the symbol for **drip** or **drop**
\drɪp\ a tiny amount of fluid that falls from something
"How fast is that **gtt** running?"

duodenum

\du:-'ɒ-də-nəm\ or
\du:-əʊ-'dɪ:-nəm\ the first part of the small intestine between the pylorus and the jejunum
"Bleeding ulcers can form in the **duodenum**."
duodenal (*adj.*)

durable power of attorney for healthcare (*acronym*)
\'dɪ:-pæk\ a legal document
"Determine whether or not the patient has a **DPAHC** on admission."

DPAHC

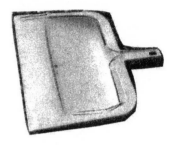

dustpan
\'dʌs-pæn\ a shovel-shaped pan for sweepings
"A **dustpan** is used with a broom."

Chapter Five

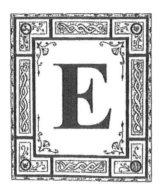

Ee \ɪ:\
The letter *E* is the fifth letter of the English alphabet.

E is for *eggs.* \egz\
"Don't put all your **eggs** in one basket."

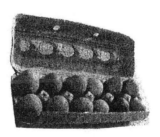

ear
\ɪə\ the organ of hearing
"Let's see if you have any wax in your
ear."

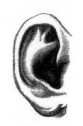

earlobe
\'ɪə ləʊb\ the bottom portion of the
outer ear
"Some young people choose to modify
their **earlobes** by stretching."
earlobes (*pl.*)

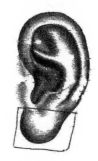

ear, nose, and throat (*abbrev.*)
\ɪ:-en-'tɪ:\ a division of medicine
"An **ENT** doctor performs
tonsillectomies."

ENT

earplugs
\'ɪə plʌgz\ a device placed in the ears to
block out sound or water
"Do you have some **earplugs** so I can
sleep?"

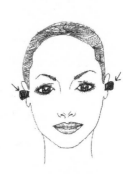

earrings
\'ɪə-rɪ:ŋz\ jewelry worn on the ears
"Dangly **earrings** are dangerous to wear
in patient-care areas."

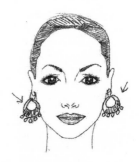

echocardiogram (*abbrev.*)
\ˈe-kəʊ\ a diagnostic test of heart
function
"A cardiac **echo** can determine the left
ventricle ejection fraction (EF)."

echo

eighth
\eɪɵ\ an ordinal number indicating the
number 8 in a series
"King Henry the **VIII (8th)** of England
had six wives."

8th

EKG stickers
\ɪ:-keɪ-ˈʤɪ: ˈstɪ-kɜ:z\ electrical
terminals or leads SYN: electrodes.
"The patient needs new **EKG stickers**."

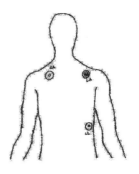

elastic bandage
\ə-ˈlæ-stɪk ˈbæn-dɪʤ\ a long, narrow
stretchy bandage used to wrap limbs or
other body parts
"A commonly used brand name for an
elastic bandage is *Ace Wrap®*
\ˈeɪs ræp\."

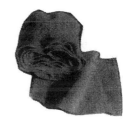

elbow
\ˈel-bəʊ\ the joint between the upper
arm and forearm
"Keep your **elbows** off the table."
elbows (*pl.*)

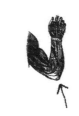

electricity
\ə-lek-'trɪ-sɪ-dɪ:\ electric current or power
"The heart runs on **electricity**."
electrical (*adj.*)

electrocardiogram (*abbrev.*)
\ɪ:-sɪ:-'ʤɪ:\ a printout of the heart's electrical conduction pattern
"Get a STAT **ECG** for any chest pain."

ECG

electrocardiogram (*abbrev.*)
\ɪ:-keɪ-'ʤɪ:\ a printout of the heart's electrical conduction pattern
"The *K* in **EKG** is from the German spelling of the word *electrocardiogram*."

EKG

electrodes
\ɪ-'lek-trəʊdz\ electrical terminals or leads
"Another name for **electrodes** is *EKG stickers*."

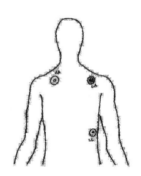

electroencephalogram (*abbrev.*)
\ɪ:-ɪ:-'ʤɪ:\ a neurologic test
"An **EEG** is ordered to analyze brain waves."

EEG

electrophysiology (*abbrev.*)
\ɪ:-'pɪ:\ the study of electrical conduction in the body
"Ablations are done in the **EP** lab."

EP

elevate
\'e-lə-veɪt\ to lift up or raise
"**Elevate** your feet when you're resting."

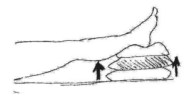

elevator
\'e-lə-veɪ-dɜ:\ a cage or platform that works to convey people or things to different levels
"Take the **elevator** up to the third floor."

emergency department (*abbrev.*)
\ɪ:-'dɪ:\ a department in the hospital
SYN: ER.
"The patient was brought to the **ED** via ambulance."

ED

emergency medical technician
\ɪ:-em-'tɪ:\ title
"**EMT**s treat patients in the field."

EMT

emergency room (*abbrev.*)
\'ɪ:-ɑ:\ a department in the hospital
SYN: ED.
"The patient was admitted from **ER**."

ER

emesis basin
\'em-ə-sɪs 'beɪ-sən\ a receptacle for expectorating or vomiting SYN: spit pan.
"An **emesis basin** is used when rinsing the mouth."

endotracheal tube (*abbrev.*)
\ɪ:-'tɪ:-tu:b\ an artificial airway
"An intubated patient has an **ET tube** in place."

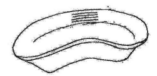

end-stage renal disease (*abbrev.*)
\ɪ:-es-ɑ:-'dɪ:\ kidney damage
"The patient with **ESRD** may have an
elevated BUN and creatinine."

ESRD

end-tidal carbon dioxide (*abbrev.*)
\ɪ:-tɪ:-sɪ:-əʊ-'tu:\ a respiratory
measurement
"Ventilated patients should have
ETCO₂ monitoring."

ETCO2

entrance
\'en-trəns\ the way in
"I'll meet you at the main **entrance**."

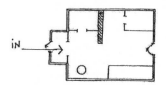

epinephrine (*abbrev.*)
\'e-pɪ:\ adrenaline
"Give one amp of **epi**."

epi

Epstein-Barr virus (*abbrev.*)
\ɪ:-bɪ:-'vɪ:\ a type of virus
"**EBV** infection is also known as
mononucleosis."

EBV

equal sign
\'ɪ:-kwəl sɑɪn\ a mathematical symbol
"One ounce = 30 ml."

=

erythrocyte sedimentation rate
(*abbrev.*)
\ɪ:-es-'ɑ:\ a hematology test
"An elevated **ESR** can reflect
inflammation."

ESR

erythromycin (*abbrev.*)
\ə-rɪ:-ərəʊ-'mɑɪ-sɪn\ an antibiotic
"**EM** is one of his allergies."

EM

erythropoietin (*abbrev.*)
\ɪ:-pɪ:-'əʊ\ a cytokine made by the kidneys
"Weekly **EPO** injections can help anemic patients manufacture more red blood cells."

EPO

esophagus
\ɪ-'sɒ-fə-gə-es\ the muscular tube that carries swallowed foods from the pharynx to the stomach
"The patient with liver cirrhosis has **esophageal** varices."
esophageal (*adj.*)

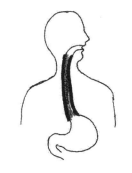

estimated blood loss (*abbrev.*)
\ɪ:-bɪ:-'el\ a calculation of blood loss
"The **EBL** in surgery was 500 ml."

EBL

estimated time of arrival (*abbrev.*)
\ɪ:-tɪ:-'eɪ\ a notice of arrival to the hospital
"An ambulance driver will give the hospital an **ETA**."

ETA

ethyl alcohol; alcoholism (*abbrev.*)
\ɪ:-tɪ:-əʊ-'eɪtʃ\ ethanol and its consumption
"*DTs* is the name for **ETOH** withdrawal symptoms."

ETOH

evaluate and treat (*abbrev.*)
\ɪ:-væl-ən-'trɪ:t\ a physician's order for rehab services
"PT/OT **E&T**."

E & T

exclamation point
\eks-clə-'meɪ-ʃən pɔɪnt\ a punctuation
mark
"An **exlcamation point** might be used
as a caution symbol."

exit
\'ek-zɪt\ the way out
"The **exit** signs are usually lit up so you
can find them."

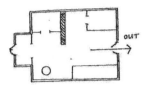

extend
\eks-'tend\ to straighten or stretch out
SYN: straighten. ANT: flex, bend.
"He cannot **extend** his arm due to the
contractures."
extension (*n.*)

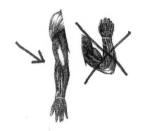

extended-spectrum beta-lactamase
(*abbrev.*)
\ɪ:-es-bɪ:-'el\ an antibiotic-resistant
microorganism
"The patient is in isolation for **ESBL** in
the blood."

ESBL

eyeballs
\'ɑɪ-bɒlz\ the organs of visions
"Removal of the **eyeballs** is called
enucleation."

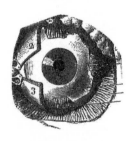

eyebrows
\'ɑɪ-brɑʊz\ the arch over the eyes
"The **eyebrows** can convey emotion."

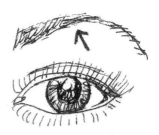

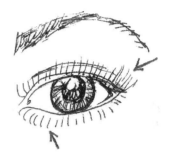

eyelashes
\'ɑɪ-læ-ʃəz\ stiff hairs on the margins of
the eyelids
"Mascara is used to darken the
eyelashes."

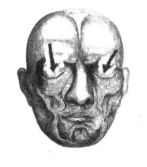

eyelids
\'ɑɪ-lɪdz\ the protective skin that covers
the eyes
"Eyeshadow is used to color the
eyelids."

Chapter Six

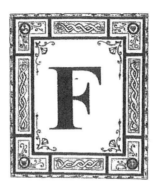

Ff \ef\
The letter *F* is the sixth letter of the English alphabet.

F is for *fish*. \fɪʃ\
"There's more than one **fish** in the sea."

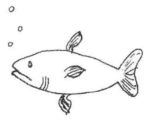

facial droop

\'feɪ-ʃəl druːp\ a weakness or paralysis of the muscles in one half of the face
"**Facial droop** is one symptom of a CVA."

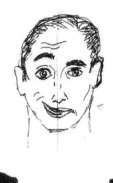

fallopian tubes

\fə-'ləʊ-pɪː-ən tuːbz\ the hollow structure that conveys the ovum from the ovary to the uterus
"A tubal ligation severs the **fallopian tubes**."

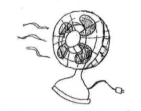

fan

\fæn\ an instrument for producing a current of air
"Cooling measures include the use of a **fan**."

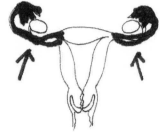

farina

\fə-'rɪː-nə\ a fine meal of vegetable matter; a hot breakfast cereal SYN: wheat cereal.
"Your breakfast choices are oatmeal, **farina**, or cold cereal."

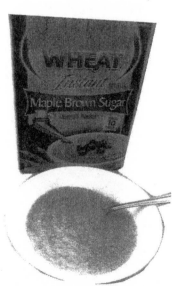

feather
\'fe-ɵɜ:\ a plume from a bird
"A great achievement may be called *a feather in your cap*."

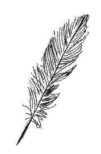

February (*abbrev.*)
\'fe-bru:-eɵ-ɪ:\ the second month of the year
"**Feb.** 14 is Valentine's Day."

Feb.

fecal occult blood test (*abbrev.*)
\'fɪ:-kəl ə-'kʌlt blʌd test\ a test for blood in the stool
"Another name for **FOBT** is *guaiac* \'gwɑɪ-æk\."

FOBT

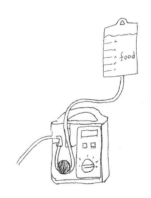

feeding pump
\'fɪ:-dɪ:ŋ pʌmp\ a device that delivers liquid nutrition into a feeding tube
"NG bolus feedings are given with a **feeding pump**."

felt-tip pen
\felt tɪp 'pen\ a writing implement with a soft tip that distributes the ink
"A commonly used brand name for **felt-tip pen** is *Sharpie®* \ʃɑ:-pɪ\."

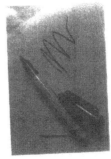

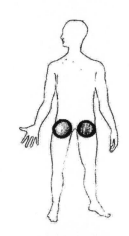

femoral
\'fem-ə-rəl\ pertaining to the femur
"He has a **femoral** central line in place."

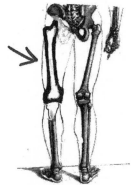

femur
\'fɪ:-mɜ:\ the thigh bone
"The **femur** is the largest bone in the human body."

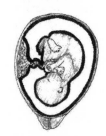

fetus
\'fɪ:-dəs\ a baby in the womb
"**Fetal** heart tones can be heard with a doppler."
fetal (*adj.*)

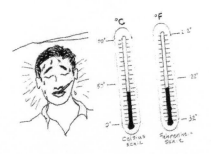

fever
\'fɪ:-vɜ:\ an elevated body temperature
"A **fever** may indicate infection."

fever of unknown origin (*abbrev.*)
\'fiː-vɜː ʌv 'ʌn-nəʊn 'ɔː-ə-dʒən\ a
condition of elevated body temperature
"The patient was admitted with a
diagnosis of **FUO**."

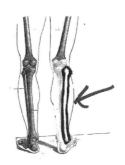

fibula
\'fɪb-juː-lə\ the smaller bone of the
lower leg
"The **fibula** is the smaller bone of the
lower leg."

fifth
\fɪθ\ an ordinal number indicating
number 5 in a series
"There are many fancy stores on **5th**
Avenue in New York City."

finger
\'fɪːŋ-ɜː\ a digit of the hand
"Humans generally have ten **fingers**."
fingers (*pl.*)

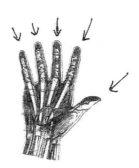

fingernail
\'fɪŋ-ɜː-neɪl\ the hard portion of the
epidermis at the end of the finger
"Healthcare workers should keep their
fingernails short and clean."
fingernails (*pl.*)

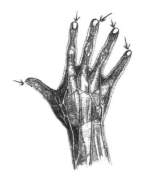

finger-stick blood sugar (*abbrev.*)
\'fɪŋ-ɜ: stɪk 'blʌd ʃʊ-gɜ:\ a blood
glucose measurement
"**FSBS**s are often done before meals
and at bedtime."

fire
\'faɪ-ɜ:\ combustion manifested in light,
flame and heat
"In the event of **fire**, use the stairs
instead of the elevator."

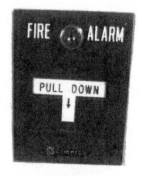

fire alarm
\'faɪ-ɜ: ə-'lɑ:m\ a signal to warn people
of a fire
"The **fire alarms** are tested
periodically."
fire alarms (*pl.*)

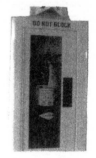

fire extinguisher
\'faɪ-ɜ: eks-'tɪŋ-wɪ-ʃɜ:\ a portable
cylinder containing chemicals to put out
a fire
"OSHA requires that employees
can easily find and operate a **fire
extinguisher** in their workplace if
necessary."

first
\fɜ:st\ an ordinal number indicating
number 1 in a series
"You will be nervous when giving your
1st IM injection."

1st

fist
\fɪst\ the hand clenched with the fingers folded into the palms
"He was mad and shook his **fist** at me."

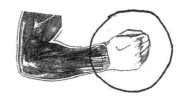

flashlight
\'flæʃ-lɑɪt\ a small portable electric light
"A **flashlight** is used to check a patient's pupil reaction."

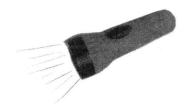

flex
\fleks\ to contract or bend SYN: bend. opp. of extend, straighten.
"Can you **flex** your feet, please?"

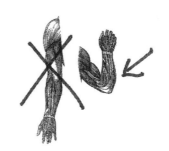

flowers
\'flɑʊ-ɜ:z\ the ornamental and fragrant blossoms of a plant
"**Flowers** are contraindicated for the neutropenic patient."

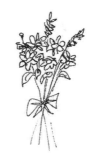

flow meter
\fləʊ 'mɪ:-dɜ:\ an instrument for measuring the flow of oxygen
SYN: oxygen meter.
"A pediatric **flow meter** will help you regulate the smaller dose of FiO_2."

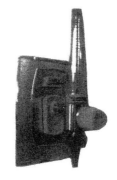

follow-up (*abbrev.*)
\'fɒ-leʊ-ʌp\ a future plan of care
"**F/U** with PCP in one week."

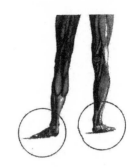

foot
\fʊt\ the body part attached to the leg at
the ankle
"Can you push your **foot** against my
hand?"
feet (*pl.*).

foot of bed
\fʊt-ʌv-'bed\ the lower portion of the
bed
"The abbreviation for **foot of bed** is
FOB."

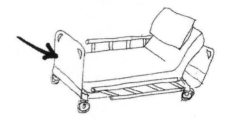

forearm
\'fɔ:-ɑ:m\ the lower part of the arm
between the elbow and the wrist
"The IV is in the left **forearm**."

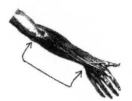

forearm (*abbrev.*)
\'fɔ:-ɑ:m\ forearm
"The IV is in his left **FA**."

FA

forehead
\'fɔ:-hed\ the front part of the head
above the eyes
"I'm going to put this thermometer on
your **forehead**."

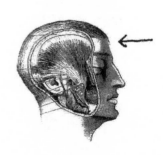

fork
\fɔ:k\ a utensil for eating
"A **fork** may be dangerous for a patient
who is hallucinating."

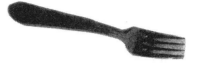

4 × 4
\'fɔ:-baɪ-fɔ:\ a piece of sterile gauze
approximately four inches square
"Use **4 × 4s** for that wet-to-dry
dressing."

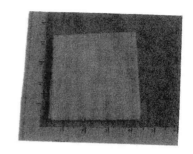

fourth
\fɔ:ə\ an ordinal number indicating
number 4 in a series
"Picnics and fireworks are part of the
4th of July."

4th

**fractional concentration of inspired
oxygen** (*abbrev.*)
\ef-aɪ-əʊ-'tu:\
"**FiO$_2$** is the amount of oxygen a patient
is receiving."

FiO2

fracture
\'fræk-ʃɜ:\ a broken bone SYN: break.
"That patient needed surgery to repair
his tibia **fracture**."

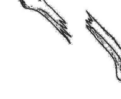

fresh frozen plasma (*abbrev.*)
\ef-ef-'pɪ:\ a blood component (serum)
"**FFP** is given to help with clotting
factors."

FFP

Friday (*abbrev.*)
\'frɑɪ-deɪ\ the sixth day of the week
"TGIF means *thank God it's* **Fri.**"

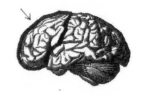

frontal lobe
\'frʌn-təl ləʊb\ the front part of the
cerebral cortex
"An injury to the **frontal lobe** can cause
a change in personality."

frown
\fraʊn\ a disapproving or unpleasant
facial expression
"The corners of the mouth point down
in a **frown**."

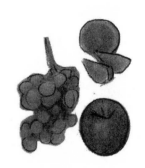

fruit
\fru:t\ the usually edible reproductive
body of a seed plant
"Fresh **fruit** is condraindicated for the
neutropenic patient."

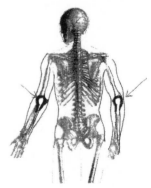

funny bone
\'fʌ-nɪ: bəʊn\ the ulnar nerve at the
elbow
"Ow! I banged my **funny bone**."

Chapter Seven

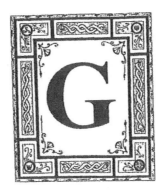

Gg \dʒɪː\
The letter *G* is the seventh letter of the English alphabet.

G is for *guitar*. \gɪ-'tɑː\
"B. B. King is a famous American **guitar** player."

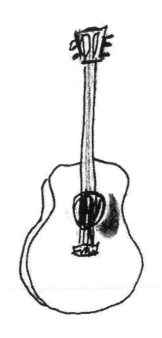

gallbladder
\gɒl ’blæ-dɜ:\ a pear-shaped sac on the underside of the liver that stores bile
“**Gallbladder** pain may mimic angina pain.”

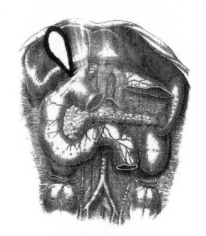

gallbladder (*abbrev.*)
\gɒl ’blæ-dɜ:\ a pear-shaped sac on the underside of the liver that stores bile
“Removal of the **GB** is called a *cholecystectomy*.”

gallon
\'gæ-lən\ a unit of volume
“One **gallon** is equal to four quarts.”

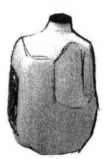

gamma
\'gæ-mə\ the third letter of the Greek alphabet
“**Gamma** globulins may be given to help boost immunity.”

gastroesophageal reflux disease
(*acronym*)
\gɜ:d\ a disorder of stomach acid
“The patient takes an acid blocker for his **GERD**.”

gauze
\gɒz\ a loosely woven cotton surgical dressing
"Dry **gauze** is one type of wound dressing."

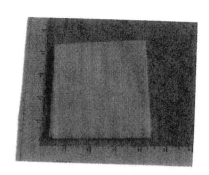

general practitioner (*abbrev.*)
\dʒɪ-ˈpɪ:\ a title
"Who is the patient's **GP**?"

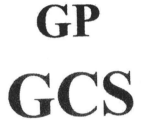

Glasgow Coma Scale (*abbrev.*)
\dʒɪ-sɪ:-ˈes\ a neurological assessment
"A healthy **GCS** score is 15."

glass
\glæs\ a usually clear drinking container
"Can I have a **glass** of water to swallow my pills with?"

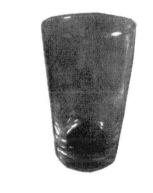

glasses
\ˈglæ-səz\ lenses worn to aid vision
"Many people cannot read without **glasses**."

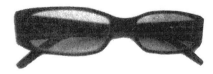

glomerular filtration rate (*abbrev.*)
\dʒɪ:-ef-ˈɑ:\ a measure of kidney function
"Check the **GFR** before doing the CT scan."

gloves
\glʌvz\ protective hand covering
"This procedure requires sterile **gloves**."

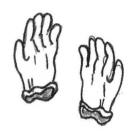

gluteal
\'glu:-dɪ:-əl\ of or related to the gluteus
muscles
"IM injections are frequently given in a
gluteal site."

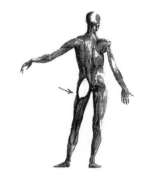

golf ball
\'gɒlf bɒl\ a small hard dimpled ball
used in golf
"I feel like there's a **golf ball** stuck in
my throat."

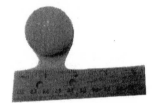

gonads
\'gəʊ-nædz\ reproductive glands, such
as the ovary or testis
"Pituitary hormones are involved in
regulating the activity of the **gonads**."

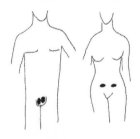

graduate
\'græ-dʒu:-ɪt\ a container for measuring
liquids
"A **graduate** holds one liter."

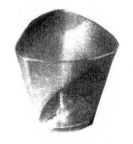

symbol for **greater than**
\'greɪ-dɜ: ðæn\ a mathematical symbol
"Keep SBP > 90."

grimace
\'grɪ-məs\ a facial expression of digust
or disapproval
"**Grimacing** may be an indication of
distress or pain."

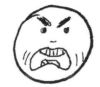

grin
\grɪn\ to show the teeth
"A **grin** may be a sign of happiness."

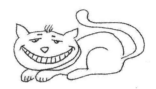

grip
\grɪp\ to seize or hold firmly with the
hand
"Compare bilateral **grip** strength."

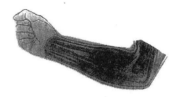

groin
\grɔɪn\ the depression between the thigh
and the trunk SYN: crotch.
"The patient has a **groin** rash."

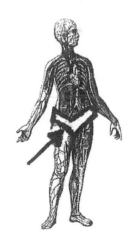

gum
\gʌm\ a sweetened and flavored material
designed for chewing SYN: chewing
gum.
"Do you have a piece of **gum**?"

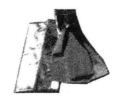

gums

\gʌmz\ the mucosal tissue covering the alveolar processes of the mandible and maxilla
"Check the **gums** for bleeding while the patient is on blood thinners."

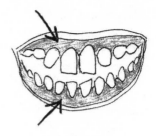

gun

\gʌn\ a portable firearm
"It is illegal to bring a **gun** to the hospital."

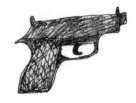

Chapter Eight

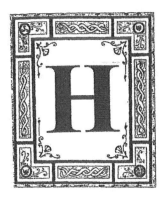

Hh \eɪtʃ\
The letter *H* is the eighth letter of the English alphabet.

H is for *heart*. \hɑːt\
"'I Left My **Heart** in San Francisco' is sung by Tony Bennett."

hairbrush
\'heə brʌʃ\ a utensil with bristles for smoothing the hair SYN: brush.
"Most women prefer a **hairbrush** for their hair instead of a comb."

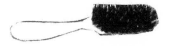

hallux
\'hæl-əks\ the first or great toe SYN: big toe.
"The word *hallux* is rarely used in general conversation to describe the big toe."

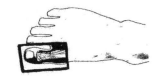

hallway
\'hɒl-weɪ\ a passageway or corridor
"**Hallways** are kept clear in case of emergency."
hallways (*pl.*)

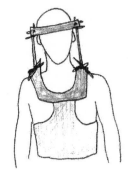

halo
\'heɪ-ləʊ\ an apparatus used to immobilize the neck due to injury; a ring around the head
"The patient was in a **halo** after his cervical spine fracture."

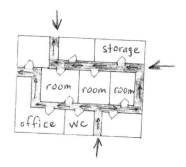

hammer
\'hæ-mɜ:\ a tool for driving nails
"He got a hematoma from getting hit in the head with a **hammer**."

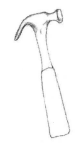

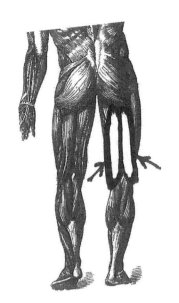

hamstrings
\'hæm-strɪ:ŋz\ any of the three muscles
on the posterior aspect of the thighs
"Do some **hamstring** stretches before
working out."
hamstring (*s.*)

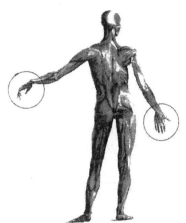

hand
\hænd\ the body part attached to the
forearm at the wrist
"Here's something to wash your **hands**
before breakfast."
hands (*pl.*)

handheld nebulizer (*abbrev.*)
\eɪʧ-eɪʧ-'en\ a device that delivers mist
SYN: nebulizer.
"**HHN** treatments are ordered every
four hours."

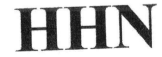

happy face
\'hæ-pɪ: feɪs\ a cartoon image of a
smiling face SYN: smiley face.
"She always draws a little **happy face**
on her notes."

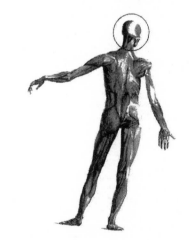

hard of hearing (*abbrev.*)
\hɑ:d-ʌv-'hɪə-ɪ:ŋ\ a designation of
hearing loss
"The patient is **HOH**, and he doesn't
have his hearing aids."

HOH

hat
\hæt\ a plastic receptacle for measuring
urine
"I put a **hat** in the toilet for I&O."

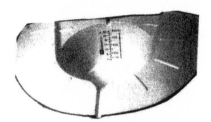

head
\hed\ the part of the body that contains
the brain and sensory organs
"The adult human **head** weighs about
ten pounds."

head of bed
\hed-ʌv-'bed\ the upper portion of the
bed
"The abbreviation for **head of bed** is
HOB."

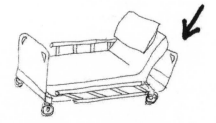

headphones
\'hed-fəʊnz\ an earphone held over the
ear by a band worn on the head
"Do you have any **headphones** for this
TV?"

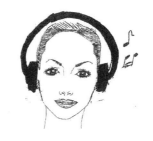

**Health Insurance Portability and
Accountability Act** (*acronym*)
\'hɪ-pə\ a set of laws
"**HIPAA** laws dictate rules about patient
confidentiality."

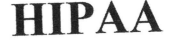

hearing aid
\'hɪə-ɪːŋ eɪd\ an electronic device worn
to amplify sound
"Care should be taken to protect a
patient's **hearing aids**."
aids (*pl.*)

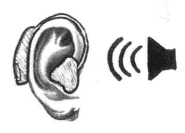

heart
\hɑːt\ the muscular pump of the
circulatory system
"**Heart** disease will become more
common as the population ages."

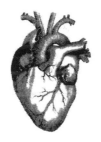

heel
\hɪːl\ the rounded posterior portion of
the foot SYN: calcaneus.
"Float the patient's **heels** to prevent
pressure sores."
heels (*pl.*)

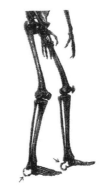

height (*abbrev.*)
\haɪt\ a measure of body length
"Document the patient's **ht.** and wt. on
admission."

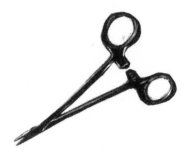

hemoglobin and hematocrit (*abbrev.*)
\eɪtʃ-ɪn-'eɪtʃ\ a hematology test
"The GI bleed patient is getting **H&Hs**
drawn Q6h."

hemostat
\'hɪː-mə-stæt\ a compressor for
controlling hemorrhage of a bleeding
vessel
SYN: clamp.
"A **hemostat** has a lock on the handles
to hold it in position."

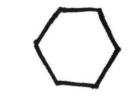

hexagon
\'heks-ə-gɒn\ a polygon of six angles
and six sides
"The holes in a bee's honeycomb are
hexagonal."
hexagonal (*adj.*)

hips
\hɪps\ the regions lateral to the pelvic
bones
"Fractured **hips** are more likely to occur
in older patients with osteoporosis."

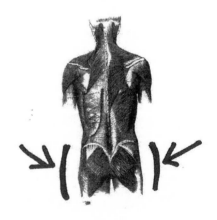

history (*abbrev.*)
\'hɪs-tɜ:-ɪ:\ an account of a patient's medical background
"The patient has a **hx** of pneumonia."

hx

history and physical (*abbrev.*)
\eɪtʃ-ɪn-'pɪ:\ a description of a patient's history and a physical examination
"Please have dictation type out the **H&P** I just dictated ASAP."

H & P

hora somni
\eɪtʃ-'es\ Latin for "at bedtime"
"Temazepam 15 mg p.o. QHS prn insomnia."

HS

hospital gown
\'hɒs-pɪ-dəl gaʊn\ a garment for patients to wear
"A **hospital gown** ties in the back."

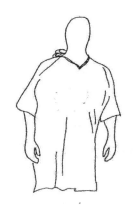

hot
\hɒt\ a condition of higher temperature
"**Hot** is the opposite of *cold*."

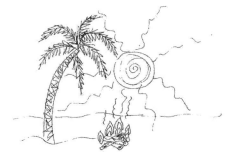

human immunodeficiency virus
(*abbrev.*)
\eɪʧ-ɑɪ-'vɪ:\ a type of virus
"AIDS results from being infected with
HIV."

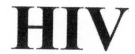

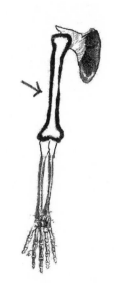

humerus
\'hju:-mə-rəs\ the bone of the upper arm
"The patient has a fractured right
humerus."

symbol for **hydrogen peroxide**
\'hɑɪ-drʌ-ʤən pɜ:-'ɒk-sɑɪd\ a
germicidal solution
"Clean the tracheostomy with
half-strength H_2O_2."

$$H2O2$$

hypertension (*abbrev.*)
\hɑɪ-pɜ:-'ten-ʃən\ a condition of high
blood pressure
"The patient's health history includes
HTN, AF, and CHF."

$$HTN$$

Chapter Nine

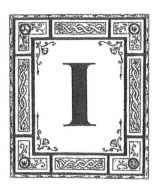

Ii \ɑɪ\
The letter *I* is the ninth letter of the English alphabet.

I is for *ice cream.* \'ɑɪs krɪ:m\
"I scream, you scream, we all scream for **ice cream!**"

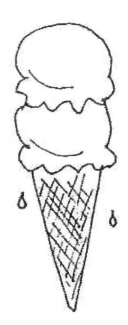

idiopathic thrombocytopenia purpura
(*abbrev.*)
\ɑɪ-tɪː-'pɪː\ a disorder of blood clotting
"One symptom of **ITP** is small bruises
on the skin."

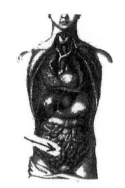

ileum
\'ɪl-ɪː-əm\ a portion of the small
intestine between the jejunum and
cecum
"The patient has some kind of bowel
obstruction in the **ileum**."
ileal (*adj.*)

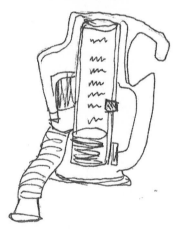

incentive spirometer
\ɪn-'sen-tɪv spɜː-'ɒ-mə-dɜː\ a tool used
to encourage patients to practice deep
breathing
"An **incentive spirometer** is ordered
post-op."

incentive spirometer (*abbrev.*)
\ɑɪ-'es\ a tool used to encourage
patients to practice deep breathing
"Encourage **IS** use 10×/hr. while
awake."

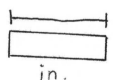

inch
\ɪntʃ\ a unit of length
"One **inch** equals 2.5 centimeters."

incision
\ɪn-'sɪ-ʒən\ a surgical cut
"An **incision** is a type of cut."

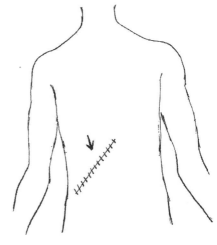

incision and drainage (*abbrev.*)
\aɪ-ən-'dɪː\ a surgical procedure
"An abscess may be treated by **I&D**."

symbol for **increase**
\ɪn-'krɪːs\ to make greater; augment
"**Increase** the frequency of HHNs to
Q2h."

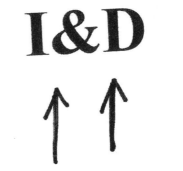

index finger
\'ɪn-deks 'fɪŋ-ʒː\ the second finger of
the hand
"The **index finger** may also be called
the *pointer* finger."

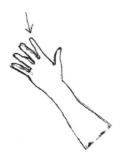

information technology (*abbrev.*)
\aɪ-'tɪː\ computer and information
systems
"Computer specialists provide **IT**
support."

inhaler
\ɪn-'heɪl-ɜ:\ a device for administering
medicines by inhalation
"He has been using his **inhaler** for
asthma attacks."

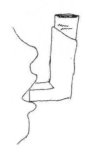

instep
\'ɪn-step\ the dorsal surface of the foot
"The metatarsals are inflamed causing
pain in the **instep** area."

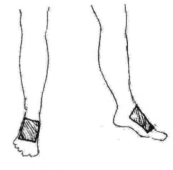

insulin syringe
\'ɪn-sə-lən sə-'rɪndʒ\ a syringe
designed to measure and administer
insulin subcutaneously
"An **insulin syringe** has an orange cap
and a fine needle."

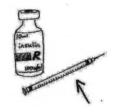

insulin-dependent diabetes mellitus
(abbrev.)
\aɪ-dɪ:-dɪ:-'em\ a disorder of blood
glucose regulation
"Type I diabetes is a form of **IDDM**."

IDDM

intake and output *(abbrev.)*
\aɪ-ɪn-'əʊ\ the measurement of fluids
consumed and excreted
"Careful **I&O** is necessary to monitor
fluid balance."

I & O

intensive care unit (*abbrev.*)
\ɑɪ-sɪː-'juː\ a department in the hospital
"Transfer the patient to **ICU** for closer
observation."

ICU

internal jugular (*abbrev.*)
\ɑɪ-'dʒeɪ\ a vein in the neck that
receives blood from the brain
"The IV site is an **IJ** line."

IJ

intestines
\ɪn-'tes-tɪnz\ the portion of the
alimentary canal that extends from the
pylorus of the stomach to the anus
"Another name for **intestines** is *gut*."
intestinal (*adj.*)

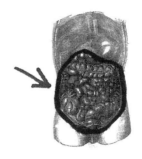

intra-aortic balloon pump (*abbrev.*)
\ɪn-trə-eɪ-'ɔː-dɪk bʌ-'luːn pʌmp\
a mechanical device that increases
coronary blood flow
"An **IABP** is used to treat heart failure."

IABP

intracranial pressure (*abbrev.*)
\ɑɪ-sɪː-'pɪː\ the pressure inside the skull
"**ICP** is monitored on patients with head
injuries."

ICP

intramuscular (*abbrev.*)
\ɑɪ-'em\ a route for injections
"Demerol 50 mg **IM** Q4h prn pain."

IM

intravenous (*abbrev.*)
\ɑɪ-'vɪː\ a route for medication
administration
"He has a 20g **IV** in the left wrist."

IV

intravenous fluids (*abbrev.*)
\ɑɪ-vɪ:-'flu:-ɪdz\ fluids administered
into a vein
"Cont. **IVF** tonight for gentle
hydration."

IVF

symbol for the element **iodine**
\'ɑɪ-ə-dɑɪn\ refer to the periodic table
of the elements
"Some patients are allergic to topical
iodine."

I

symbol for the element **iron**
\'ɑɪ-3:n\ refer to the periodic table of
the elements
"**Iron** supplements are sometimes used
to treat anemia."

Fe

irritable bowel syndrome (*abbrev.*)
\ɑɪ-bɪ:-'es\ a gastrointestinal disorder
"**IBS** can cause chronic cramping and
diarrhea."

IBS

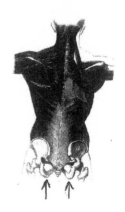

ischial tuberosity
\'ɪ-ʃɪ:-əl tu:-b3:-'ɒ-sə-dɪ:\ a prominence
on the lower edge of the pelvis that
supports a person's weight when sitting
"Prolonged bicycle riding may cause
pain in the **ischial tuberosity** area."

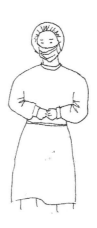

isolation gown
\ɑɪ-səʊ-'leɪ-ʃən gɑʊn\ a gown worn
over the clothes in the hospital to
prevent contamination
"**Isolation gowns** are designed to be
nonpermeable."
gowns (*pl.*)

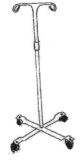

IV pole
\ɑɪ-'vɪ: pəʊl\ a stand to hold an IV
"The IV and feeding pumps attach to
the **IV poles**."
poles (*pl.*)

Chapter Ten

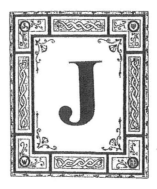

Jj \dʒeɪ\
The letter *J* is the tenth letter of the English alphabet.

J is for *jewelry*. \'juːl-rɪː\
"Shiny **jewelry** is sometimes called *bling*."

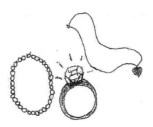

jacket
\'dʒæ-kət\ an outer garment for the
upper body
"A **jacket** may be worn in cool
weather."

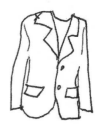

Jackson-Pratt bulb drain (*abbrev.*)
\dʒeɪ-'pɪ:\ a device that applies suction
to a drain
"Empty **JP** Q8h and record output."

JP

January (*abbrev.*)
\'dʒæn-ju:-eə-ɪ:\ the first month of the
year
"**Jan.** 1 is New Year's Day."

Jan.

jejunostomy tube (*abbrev.*)
\'dʒeɪ-tu:b\ a type of feeding tube
"The patient has an established **J-tube**
for feedings."

J-tube

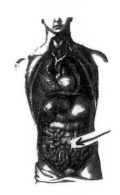

jejunum
\dʒə-'dʒu:-nəm\ the middle portion
of the small intestine, between the
duodenum and the ileum
"A J-tube extends into the **jejunum**."

**Joint Commission on the
Accreditation of Healthcare
Organizations** (*acronym*)
\dʒeɪ-sɪ:-eɪ-eɪtʃ-'əʊ\ a hospital
accreditation organization
"**JCAHO** prefers to be called the *Joint
Commission*."

JCAHO

jugular vein
\'ʤʌg-ju:-lɜ: veɪn\ any of the two pairs of bilateral veins that return blood to the heart from the head and neck
"Check the **jugular vein** for distention."

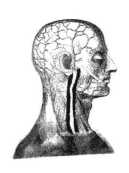

jugular venous distention (*abbrev.*)
\ʤeɪ-vɪ:-'dɪ:\ increased pressure in the jugular veins
"**JVD** can indicate fluid overload."

JVD

July
\ʤə-'laɪ\ the seventh month of the year
"**July** 4 is Independence Day."

July

June
\ʤu:n\ the sixth month of the year
"Father's Day is in **June**."

June

Chapter Eleven

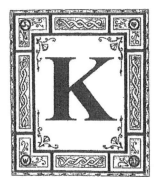

Kk \keɪ\
The letter *K* is the eleventh letter of the English alphabet.

K is for *kangaroo*. \kæŋ-ə-'ru:\
"The **kangaroo** is a symbol of Australia."

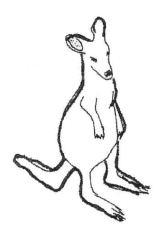

Kelly clamp
\'ke-lɪ: klæmp\ a curved metal surgical
clamp used for grasping or compressing
"A **Kelly clamp** is a type of curved
hemostat."

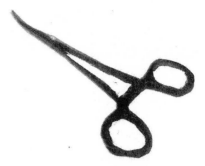

ketchup
\'ke-ʧəp\ a seasoned pureed condiment
made from tomatoes
"Fried potatoes are often eaten with
ketchup."

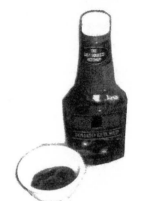

kidneys
\'kɪd-nɪ:z\ two organs situated at the
back of the abdominal cavity that filter
the blood and form urine
"The **kidneys** filter the blood."

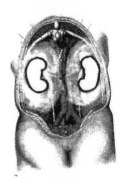

kidneys, ureters, and bladder
(*abbrev.*)
\keɪ-ju:-'bɪ:\ a type of radiologic view
"A **KUB** is an x-ray of the abdomen."

KUB

knee
\nɪ:\ the articulations formed by the distal femur, proximal tibia, and the patella
"**Knee**-replacement surgery is easier than it used to be."

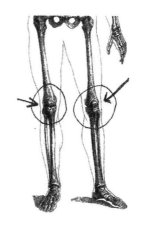

kneecap
\'nɪ:-kæp\ patella
"I keep banging my **kneecaps** on the corner of this file cabinet."
kneecaps (*pl.*)

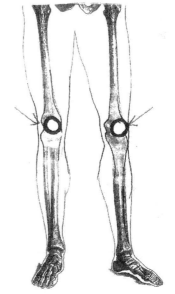

knife
\nɑɪf\ a cutting instrument consisting of a blade attached to a handle
"Silverware usually includes a **knife**, fork, and spoon."
knives (*pl.*).

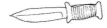

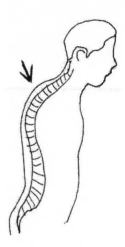

kyphosis
\kɑɪ-'fəʊ-sɪs\ an exaggeration of the posterior curve of the thoracic spine "Severe osteoporosis can cause a **kyphosis.**"

Chapter Twelve

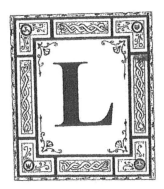

Ll \el\
The letter *L* is the twelfth letter of the English alphabet.

L is for *lightbulb*. \'laɪt-bʌlb\
"Thomas Edison's work helped develop the modern **lightbulb**."

labor and delivery (*abbrev.*)
\el-ən-'dɪ:\ a department in the hospital
SYN: OB.
"The **L&D** rooms are big and
comfortable for the family to stay in."

L & D

laceration
\læ-sɜ:-'eɪ-ʃən\ a wound or irregular
tear of the flesh
"Another word for **laceration** is *cut*."

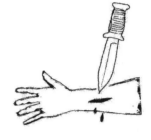

lactate dehydrogenase (*abbrev.*)
\el-dɪ:-'eɪtʃ\ an enzyme in the body
"Pleural fluid and CSF will often be
checked for **LDH** levels."

LDH

lactated Ringer's solution (*abbrev.*)
\el-'ɑ:\ an intravenous solution
"**LR** is often given in the OR."

LR

ladder
\'læ-dɜ:\ a structure for climbing up
and down
"It's bad luck to walk under a **ladder**."

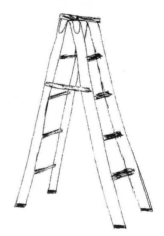

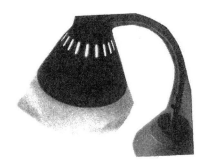

lamp
\læmp\ a device for producing light
"The **lamp** needs a new lightbulb."

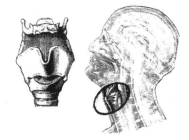

larynx
\'leə-ɪːnks\ an organ at the upper end
of the trachea that is part of the airway
and vocal apparatus SYN: voice box,
Adam's apple.
"Loss of the voice due to a viral
infection that has inflamed the **larynx** is
called *laryngitis*."
laryngeal (*adj.*)

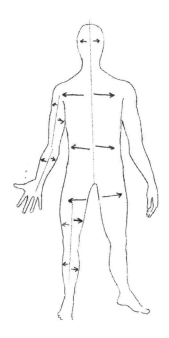

lateral
\'læ-dɜː-əl\ away from the center of the
body SYN: side.
"There is a pressure sore on the right
lateral mallelolus."

lateral (*abbrev.*)
\læt\ away from the center of the body;
side
"Get a PA and **lat** CXR after the
pacemaker is placed."

lat

left anterior descending artery
(*abbrev.*)
\el-eɪ-'dɪ:\ one of the coronary arteries
"The patient with an **LAD** occlusion
needs a CABG."

LAD

left main artery (*abbrev.*)
\left meɪn\ one of the coronary arteries
"His heart cath showed an **LM**
occlusion."

LM

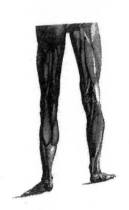

legs
\legz\ the lower extremities
"Your **legs** may feel weak from being in
bed for so long."

symbol for less than
\'les ðæn\ a mathematical symbol
"Keep the SBP < 160."

level
\'le-vəl\ having no part higher than the
other
"**Level** is the opposite of *uneven*."

level of consciousness (*abbrev.*)
\el-əʊ-'sɪ:\ a neurological assessment
"The patient was admitted with altered
LOC."

LOC

lidocaine (*abbrev.*)
\'lɑɪ-dəʊ\ a medication.
"I need some SQ **lido** for the sutures."

lido

life support
\'lɑɪf sə-pɔ:t\ the use of any technique,
therapy, or device to assist in sustaining
life SYN: respirator, ventilator.
"The patient requests no mechanical **life
support**."

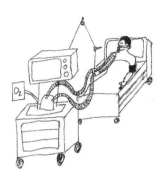

lighter
\'lɑɪ-dʒɜ:\ a device used for lighting
cigars, cigarettes or pipes
"The patient's cigarettes and **lighter**
were placed in the hospital safe."

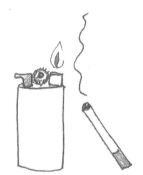

lip balm
\lɪp bɒlm\ a healing ointment for the
lips
"Use only non-petroleum **lip balm** in
the hospital when oxygen is in use."

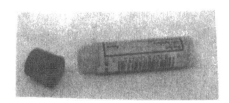

lips
\lɪps\ the soft, external structures that
form the boundary of the mouth
"When the **lips** turn blue from lack of
oxygen, it is called *cyanosis*."

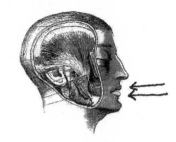

lipstick
\'lɪp-stɪk\ decorative coloring for the
lips
"Please remove your **lipstick** when
practicing on the CPR mannequins."

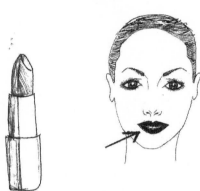

liver
\'lɪ-vɜ:\ the largest solid organ of the
body situated on the right side below the
diaphragm; it secretes bile and is the site
of numerous metabolic functions
"Alcohol consumption can damage the
liver."

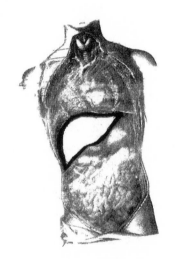

liver function tests (*abbrev.*)
\el-ef-'tɪ:z\ blood chemistry levels that
reflect liver function
"A liver ultrasound was ordered for
elevated **LFTs**."

LFT's

lobster
\'lɒb-stɜ:\ any of a family of large
edible marine decapod crustaceans
"**Lobster** is one type of shellfish."

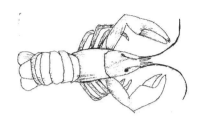

Lopez valve
\'ləʊ-pez vælv\ a three-way stopcock
that attaches to an NGT tube
"Save the adaptor at the end of the
Lopez valve in case you start tube
feedings."

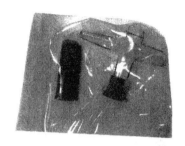

lower extremities (*abbrev.*)
\'ləʊ-ɜ: eks-'tre-mɪ-dɪ:z\ SYN: legs.
"Place the SCDs on the bilat. **LEs**."

LE's

low intermittent suction (*abbrev.*)
\ləʊ ɪn-tɜ:-'mɪ-tənt 'sʌk-ʃən\
"NGT to **LIS**."

LIS

Luer lock
\'lʊə-lɒk\ a type of threaded adaptor
that ensures a secure connection;
syringe
"A **Luer lock** syringe is used to draw
from an IV line port."

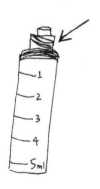

lumbar puncture

\'lʌm-bɑ: 'pʌnk-ʧɜ:\ the process of
entering the subarachnoid space to
obtain cerebrospinal fluid SYN: spinal
tap.
"A **lumbar puncture** is indicated for
fever and severe head and neck pain."

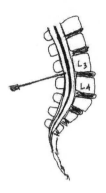

lumbar puncture (*abbrev.*)

\el-'pɪ:\ SYN: spinal tap.
"The best patient position for an **LP** is
lateral recumbent with the knees pulled
to the chest."

lungs

\lʌŋz\ the organs of respiration
contained within the pleural cavity
"A distended abdomen can prevent
adequate expansion of the **lungs**."

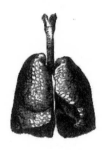

Chapter Thirteen

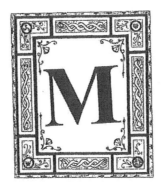

Mm \em\
The letter *M* is the thirteenth letter of the English alphabet.

M is for *moon.* \muːn\
"'**Moon** River' is a famous song by Mancini and Mercer."

the symbol for the **magnesium** ion
\mæg-'nɪ:-zɪ:-əm\ a chemical element
in the body
"The patient was having a lot of PVCs
so we checked a **Mg++** level."

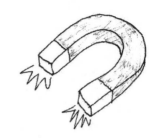

magnet
\'mæg-net\ a body having the property
of attracting iron and producing a
magnetic field external to itself
"A powerful **magnet** can disrupt
pacemaker function."

magnetic resonance angiography
(*abbrev.*)
\em-ɑ:-'eɪ\ a type of diagnostic image
"An **MRA** can detect vascular
abnormalities."

magnetic resonance imaging (*abbrev.*)
\em-ɑ:-'ɑɪ\ a type of diagnostic image
"The **MRI** machine has a powerful
magnetic field."

magnifying glass
\'mæg-nɪ-fɑɪ-ɪ:ŋ glæs\ a lens that
makes something appear larger
"I need a **magnifying glass** to read the
writing on the label."

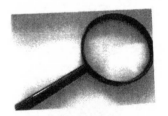

makeup
\'meɪ-kʌp\ cosmetics used to decorate
the face
"Some **makeup** can cause an allergic
reaction."

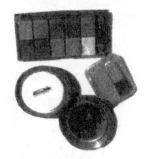

March (*abbrev.*)
\mɑːʧ\ the third month of the year
"**Mar.** 17 is St. Patrick's Day."

Mar.

mask
\mæsk\ a covering for the face that
serves as a protective barrier
"Wear a gown, gloves, and **mask** in that
isolation room."

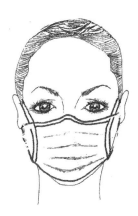

matches
\'mæ-ʧəz\ small pieces of flammable
material that burst into flames when
struck against a rough surface
"It's safe practice to not leave any
matches in a patient's room."

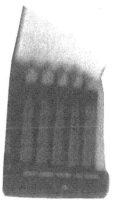

May
\meɪ:\ the fifth month of the year
"Memorial Day is on the last Monday
in **May**."

May

measles, mumps, rubella (*abbrev.*)
\em-em-'ɑː\ vaccines
"An **MMR** vaccine is routinely given to
children."

MMR

measuring tape
\'me-ʒɜ:-ɪːŋ teɪp\ a flexible intrument used to measure length
"Girth is measured with a **measuring tape**."

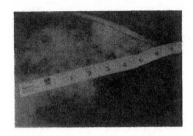

Medication Administration Record
(acronym)
\mɑ:\ or \em-eɪ-'ɑ:\ a record of drugs given
"After the meds are given, they are charted on the **MAR**."

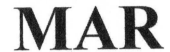

med cup
\med kʌp\ a small container used to hold and distribute medications
"Pills are administered in a **med cup**."

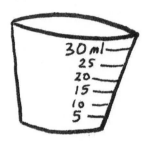

medical doctor *(title)*; **muscular dystrophy** *(abbrev.)*
\em-'dɪː\
"Some forms of **MD** diseases are hereditary."

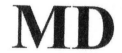

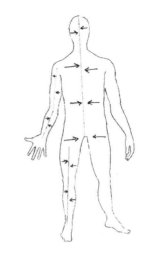

medial
\'mɪ:-dɪ:-əl\ toward the center of the body SYN: middle.
"She has an ankle fracture at the **medial** malleolus."

MedicAlert® bracelet
\'me-dɪk ə-'lɜ:t 'breɪs-lət\ a piece of jewelry that contains crucial medical information
"His **MedicAlert® bracelet** says he's a diabetic."

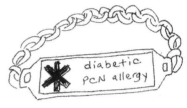

medication (*abbrev.*)
\med\ a medicinal substance; a drug
"All **meds** given in the hospital require a physician's order."
meds (*pl.*)

med

medical record number (*abbrev.*)
\'me-dɪ-kəl 're-kɜ:d 'nʌm-bɜ:\ a number assigned to each patient to preserve their records
"The **MRN** should be on the patient's nameband."

MRN

metered-dose inhaler (*abbrev.*)
\em-dɪ:-'aɪ\ a device that delivers inhaled medicines
SYN: inhaler.
"The **MDI** is ordered QID."

MDI

methicillin-resistant *Staphylococcus aureus* (*abbrev.*)
\em-ɑ:-es-'eɪ\ a type of antibiotic-resistant bacteria
"**MRSA** is a bacteria that is isolated in the hospital."

MRSA

symbol for **micrograms**
\'mɑɪ-krəʊ-græmz\ a metric unit of weight
"1 mg = 1,000 **mcg**."

mcg

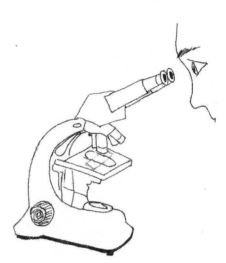

microscope
\'mɑɪ-krə-skəʊp\ an optical instrument that greatly magnifies minute objects
"A **microscope** is used to look at slides in the lab."

middle finger
\'mɪ-dəl 'fɪ:ŋ-ɜ:\ the third finger of the hand
"Extending the **middle finger** and pointing it at someone is considered a rude gesture."

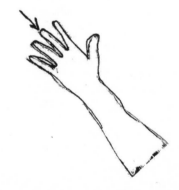

midnight (*abbrev.*)
\'mɪd-nɑɪt\ the first hour of a
twenty-four-hour-clock period
"The patient is NPO after **MN** for the
procedure tomorrow."

MN

milk
\mɪlk\ cow's milk used as a food by
humans
"Lactose-intolerant patients don't drink
milk."

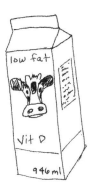

the symbol for **milliequivalents**
(*abbrev.*)
\mɪ-lɪ:-ə-'kwɪ-və-ləns\ a metric
measure of mass
"Give the patient 40 **mEq** of KCl elixir
please."

mEq

the symbol for **milligrams**
\'mɪ-lə-græmz\ a metric measure of
weight
"1 g = 1,000 **mg**."

mg

the symbol for **millimeters of mercury**
\'mɪ-lɪ-mɪ:-dɜ:z ʌv 'mɜ:k-jɜ:-ɪ:\ a unit
of pressure measurement
"Blood pressure is measured in
mmHg."

mmHg

the symbol for **millimoles**
\'mɪ-lɪ:-məʊlz\ a metric measure of
mass.
"KPO_4 is often measured in **mmol**."

mmol

mitral valve
\'mɑɪ-trəl vælv\ the heart valve
between the left atrium and left ventricle
SYN: bicuspid valve, left
atrioventricular valve.
"**Mitral valve** prolapse can be detected
on an echocardiogram."

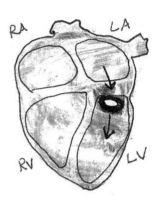

Monday (*abbrev.*)
\'mʌn-deɪ\ the second day of the week
"**Mon.** is the first day of a business
week."

Mon.

money
\'mʌ-nɪ:\ something generally accepted
as a medium of exchange; currency
"It's best to keep your **money** locked up
in the safe."

$

month (*abbrev.*)
\mʌnθ\ a period of approximately thirty
days corresponding with one moon
cycle
"F/U with MD in 6 **mo.**"

mo.

mop
\mɒp\ an implement made of absorbent
material attached to a handle and used
for cleaning floors
"Please call housekeeping to **mop** up
this spill."

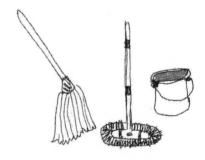

motor vehicle accident (*abbrev.*)
\em-vɪ:-'eɪ\ an abbreviation for a car
accident that resulted in an injury to the
patient
"The patient has chronic pain from a
prior **MVA**."

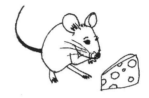

mouse
\maʊs\ rodent, genus *Mus*
"**Mouse** droppings can carry diseases."

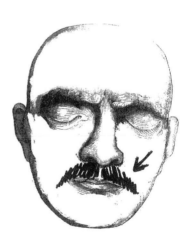

multiple sclerosis; morphine sulfate
(*abbrev.*)
\em-'es\ a neuromuscular disease; an
opioid drug
"**MS** is a degenerative disease of the
central nervous system."

mustache
\'mʌ-stæʃ\ the hair growing on the
upper lip
"He looks a lot different without his
mustache."

myocardial infarction (*abbrev.*)
\em-'aɪ\ an injury to the heart muscle
"Another name for **MI** is *heart attack*."

Chapter Fourteen

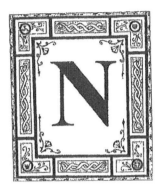

Nn \en\
The letter *N* is the fourteenth letter of the English alphabet.

N is for *north.* \nɔːə\
"The **North** Star is also called *Polaris.*"

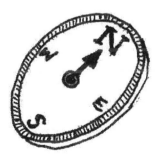

nail clippers
\neɪl 'klɪ-pɜ:z\ an instrument used to
trim finger and toenails
"Use a nail file instead of **nail clippers**
on patients who are diabetic."

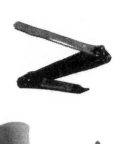

nail polish
\neɪl 'pɒ-lɪʃ\ decorative color for the
fingernails
"A pulse ox reading on a finger may
be more accurate if the **nail polish** is
removed."

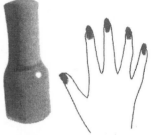

nameband
\'neɪm-bænd\ a bracelet that displays
patient identification SYN: wristband.
"The **nameband** is applied on
admission."

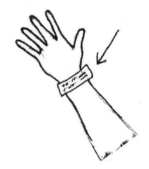

napkin
\'næp-kɪn\ a piece of material used at
the table to wipe the lips or fingers and
protect the clothes
"Paper **napkins** are disposable."
napkins (*pl.*)

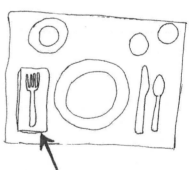

narcotics (*abbrev.*)
\nɑ:ks\ controlled substances
"All **narcs** need to be accounted for in
the hospital."

narcs

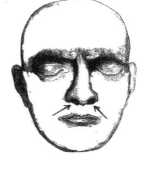

nares
\'neə-ɪ:z\ nostrils
"The patient's **nares** were swabbed for
an MRSA culture."
naris (*s.*)

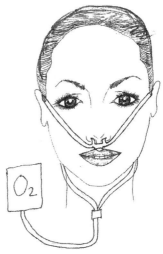

nasal cannula
\'neɪ-zəl 'kæn-ju:-lə\ plastic tubing
with prongs that delivers oxygen
through the nose
"The patient's oxygen is two liters via
nasal cannula."

nasal cannula (*abbrev.*)
\'neɪ-zəl 'kæn-ju:-lə\ plastic tubing
with prongs that delivers oxygen
through the nose
"The FiO$_2$ is 2l via **NC**."

NC

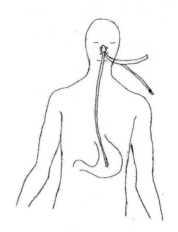

nasogastric tube
\neɪ-zəʊ-ʼgæs-trɪk tuːb\ a tube inserted through the nose that extends into the stomach
"Activated charcoal was given via **nasogastric tube**."

nasogastric tube (*abbrev.*)
\en-ʼʤɪ-tuːb\ a tube inserted through the nose that extends into the stomach
"Enteral feedings will be started via **NGT**."

NGT

navel
\ʼneɪ-vəl\ the abdominal scar from the umbilical cord SYN: umbilicus, belly button.
"It's important to keep the **navel** area clean and dry on newborns to prevent infection."

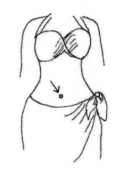

nebulizer
\ʼneb-juː-laɪ-zɜː\ an apparatus for producing a fine spray or mist
SYN: HHN.
"Albuterol is a bronchodilator given via **nebulizer**."
nebulized (*adj.*)

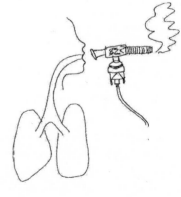

neck
\nek\ the part of the body between the head and the shoulders SYN: cervical spine.
"A *whiplash* is a type of **neck** injury."

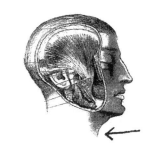

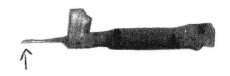

necklace
\'nek-ləs\ an ornament worn around the neck
"The patient's gold **necklace** was placed in the hospital safe."

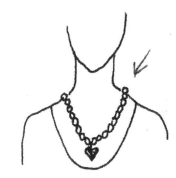

needle
\'nɪ:-dəl\ a pointed instrument used for injections or puncturing
"A 22 gauge **needle** is smaller than an 18 gauge needle."

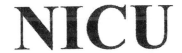

neonatal intensive care unit (*abbrev.*)
\en-ɑɪ-sɪ:-'ju:\ neonatal intensive care unit
"Premature infants are cared for in the **NICU**."

NICU

nighttime
\'naɪt-taɪm\ when the moon is up, from
dusk until dawn
"Sometimes pain is worse at
nighttime."

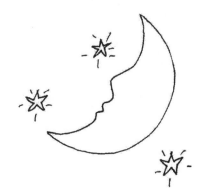

ninth
\naɪnə\ ordinal number indicating
number 9 in a series
"The **9th** inning is usually the last part
of a typical baseball game."

9th

nipple
\'nɪ-pəl\ the protuberance at the tip of
each breast
"The chest compression location on an
infant is directly below the **nipple** line."

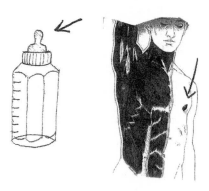

nitroglycerin (*abbrev.*)
\naɪ-troʊ-'glɪ-sɜ:-ɪn\ a medication that
dilates blood vessels
"Give **NTG** SL every 5 minutes × 3 for
chest pain."

NTG

nocturnal or **night** (*abbrev.*)
\nɒk\ the time period when the moon is
up and the sun is down
"I've been working **noc** shift."

noc

no known allergies (*abbrev.*)
\nəʊ nəʊn 'æ-lɜ:-gɪ:z\ a listing of a
patient's allergies, which are none at the
present time
"The patient's nameband says **NKA**."

NKA

**noninsulin-dependent diabetes
mellitus** (*abbrev.*)
\en-ɑɪ-dɪ:-dɪ:-'em\ a disorder of blood
glucose regulation
"**NIDDM** may be controlled with diet
and oral agents."

NIDDM

noninvasive blood pressure (*abbrev.*)
\en-ɑɪ-bɪ:-'pɪ:\ blood pressure measured
with a cuff
"Compare the art line reading with a
NIBP measurement."

NIBP

non per os (*abbrev.*)
\en-pɪ:-'əʊ\ Latin for "nothing by
mouth"
"The patient is **NPO** after midnight for
a procedure tomorrow."

NPO

nonrebreather
\nɒn-rɪ:-'brɪ:-θɜ:\ a mask with
a reservoir that delivers a high
concentration of oxygen
"The patient with a pulmonary
embolism was placed on a
nonrebreather mask."

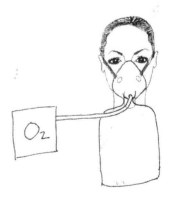

non-S-T elevation myocardial infarction (*abbrev.*)
\nɒn-'ste-mɪ:\ a type of heart attack
"Another name for a **non-STEMI** is *subendocardial myocardial infarction*."

non- STEMI

nonsteroidal anti-inflammatory drug (*abbrev.*)
\'en-seɪd\ a class of medications that includes aspirin and ibuprofen
"Taking **NSAIDS** without food can cause a gastric ulcer."

NSAID

non weight bearing (*abbrev.*)
\nɒn-'weɪt-beə-ɪ:ŋ\ a physical therapy order
"**NWB** toe-touch only on operative leg."

NWB

nose
\nəʊz\ the organ of smell and breathing
"Another name for a **nosebleed** is *epistaxis*."

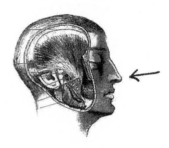

November (*abbrev.*)
\nəʊ-'vem-bɜ:\ the eleventh month of the year
"Thanksgiving is on the last Thursday in **Nov.**"

Nov.

NPH insulin
\en-pɪ:-'eɪʧ\ a type of long-acting
insulin
"**NPH** insulin will have a peak effect in
about 6-10 hours."

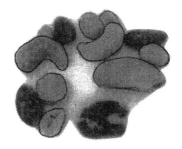

nuts
\nʌtz\ a hard-shelled dry fruit or seed
"Some patients are allergic to certain
nuts and nut oils."

Chapter Fifteen

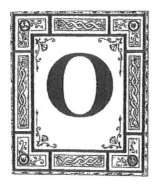

Oo \əʊ\
The letter *O* is the fifteenth letter of the English alphabet.

O is for *octagon.* \'ɒk-tə-gɒn\
"A stop sign is shaped like an **octagon**."

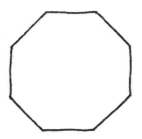

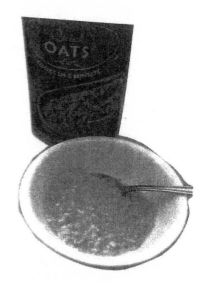

oatmeal
\'əʊt-mɪ:l\ a porridge made from ground or rolled oats
"Eating **oatmeal** may help lower cholesterol levels."

oblique
\əʊ-'blɪ:k\ at a forty-five-degree angle; inclined SYN: diagonal.
"3 views for a chest x-ray are AP, lat, and **oblique**."

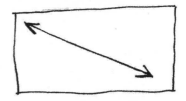

obstetrics (*abbrev.*)
\əʊ-'bɪ:\ a department in the hospital SYN: L&D.
"Babies are born in **OB**."

OB

obstructive sleep apnea (*abbrev.*)
\ʌb-'strʌk-tɪv slɪ:p 'æp-nɪ:-ə\ a disorder of breathing
"**OSA** may cause cardiomyopathy."

OSA

occipital lobe
\ɒk-'sɪ-pɪ-dəl ləʊb\ the posterior region of the cerebrum
"An injury to the **occipital lobe** can affect vision."

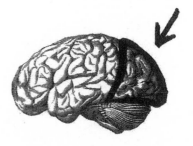

October (*abbrev.*)
\ɒk-'təʊ-bɜː\ the tenth month of the
year
"**Oct.** 31 is Halloween."

Oct.

oculus dexter
\əʊ-'dɪː\ Latin for "right eye"; overdose
"There is a patient with an opioid **OD**
in ER."

O.D.

oculus sinister
\əʊ-'es\ Latin for "left eye"
"Eye gtts **OS** TID."

O.S.

oculus uterque
\əʊ-'juː\ Latin for "each eye" (both
eyes)
"Artificial Tears **OU** prn irritation."

O.U.

the symbol for **ointment**
\'ɔɪnt-ment\ from the word *unguent*
"Apply ophthalmic **ung** OU."

ung

olecranon process
\əʊ-'lek-rə-nɒn 'prɒ-ses\ the proximal
end of the ulna that forms the bony
prominence of the elbow
"The ulnar nerve runs near the
olecranon process."

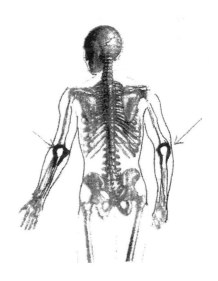

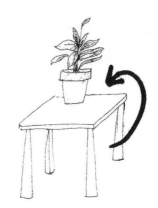

on top
\ɒn 'tɒp\ in a position above something
"The plant is **on top** of the table."

open reduction, internal fixation
(*abbrev.*)
\əʊ-ɑ:-ɑɪ-'ef\ a type of orthopedic
surgery
"The patient is going to surgery for an
ORIF of the right radial fracture."

ORIF

operating room (*abbrev.*)
\'əʊ-ɑ:\ a department in the hospital
"The **OR** temperature is cooler than
other parts of the hospital."

OR

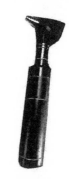

otoscope
\'əʊ-də-skəʊp\ a device for
examination of the ear
"There are disposable probe covers for
the **otoscope**."

out of bed (*abbrev.*)
\aʊt-ʌv-'bed\ an activity order; a
description of a patient's location
"The patient should get up and **OOB** for
meals."

OOB

out of control (*abbrev.*)
\ɑʊt-ʌv-kʌn-'trəʊl\ a situation or condition that is not adequately regulated
"The patient was admitted for blood glucose **OOC**."

OOC

symbol for **ounce**
\ɑʊns\ a unit of volume
"1 **oz.** equals 30 cc."

OZ.

ovaries
\'əʊ-və-rɪ:z\ the two glands in the female that produce eggs and the hormones estrogen and progesterone
"Removal of the **ovaries** is called an *oopherectomy*."
ovarian (*adj.*)

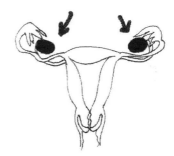

over the counter (*abbrev.*)
\əʊ-tɪ:-'sɪ:\ obtainable without a prescription
"The patient should be asked about any **OTC** medications that he or she may be taking."

OTC

oximetry
\ɒk-'sɪ-mə-trɪ:\ mesaurement of the percentage of hemoglobin in arterial blood saturated with oxygen SYN: pulse ox, SpO_2.
"The patient who has received an intrathecal injection needs to have continuous **oximetry** monitoring."

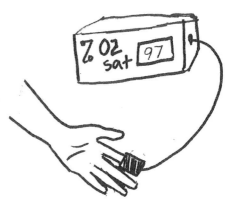

symbol for oxygen
\əʊ-'tu:\ a medicinal gas
"**Oxygen** supports combustion."

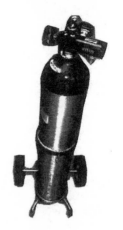

oxygen tank
\'ɒks-ɪ-ʤən tænk\ a portable metal
container for storing and delivering
oxygen
"Handle the portable **oxygen tanks** with
care."
tanks (*pl.*)

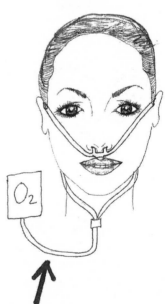

oxygen tubing
\'ɒks-ɪ-ʤən 'tu:-bɪ:ŋ\ plastic tubing
that transports oxygen to the patient
"He'll need an extension for his **oxygen
tubing** so he can get up OOB."

Chapter Sixteen

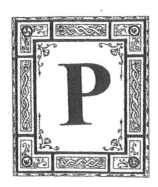

Pp \pɪ:\
The letter *P* is the sixteenth letter of the English alphabet.

P is for *pencil.* \'pen-səl\
"Scantron forms require a #2 **pencil**."

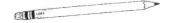

pacemaker
\'peɪs-meɪ-kɜ:\ an implanted device that
delivers electrical impulses to the heart
muscle
"He had a **pacemaker** implanted due to
episodes of profound bradycardia."

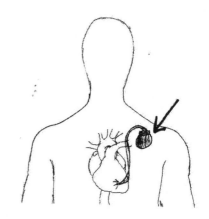

pacifier
\'pæ-sɪ-faɪ-ɜ:\ an artificial nipple given
to infants to satisfy their need to suck
"Make sure you wash the **pacifier** if it
falls on the floor."

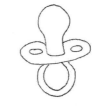

packed red blood cells (*abbrev.*)
\pɪ:-ɑ:-bɪ:-'sɪ:z\ a human blood product
"Two units of **PRBCs** were given for a
hemoglobin of 8.5."

PRBC's

palm
\pɒlm\ the anterior surface of the hand
"*Palmistry* is the art of reading hands."

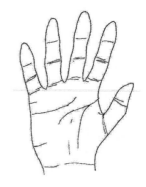

pancreas
\'pæn-krɪ:-əs\ a gland located behind
the stomach that produces digestive
enzymes and also secretes insulin and
glucagon to regulate blood sugar
"Inflammation of the **pancreas** is called
pancreatitis."

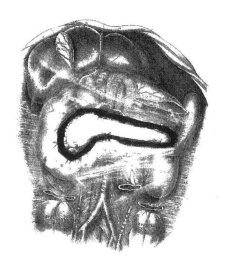

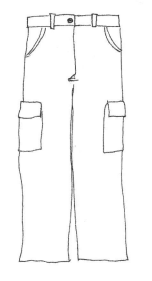

pants
\pænts\ an outer article of clothing that
covers each leg
"I want to keep my pajama **pants** on
because my legs get cold."

paper clip
\'peɪ-pɜ: klɪp\ a piece of wire bent into
flat loops to hold paper together
"Please use a **paper clip** instead of a
staple for those forms."

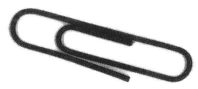

paper towels
\'peɪ-pɜ: 'taʊ-əlz\ an absorbent paper
for wiping or drying
"Our **papertowel** dispenser by the main
sink is empty."
towel (*s.*)

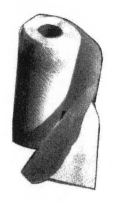

parathyroid
\peə-ə-'thaɪ-rɔɪd\ four small endocrine
glands situated close to the thyroid
that secrete parathormone to regulate
calcium and phosphorus metabolism
"She has temporary hypocalcemia
due to the shock to the **parathyroid**
glands."

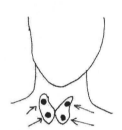

parentheses
\pə-'ren-θə-sɪ:z\ curved marks used
in writing or printing to enclose an
expression or symbol
"The full name for EGD is
written out in the **parentheses**:
(esophagogastroduodenoscopy)."

parietal lobe
\pə-'raɪ-ə-dəl ləʊb\ a portion of the
cerebrum lying beneath each parietal
bone of the skull
"The patient has a right **parietal lobe**
infarct."

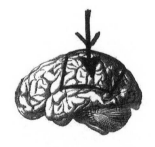

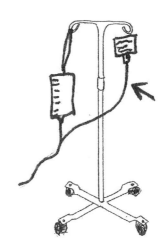

partial fill tubing
\'pɑ:-ʃʌl fɪl 'tu:-bɪ:ŋ\ a shorter piece
of IV tubing to connect intermittent
infusion bags
"I'll need some **partial fill tubing** for
the antibiotic."

patella
\pə-'te-lə\ a small bone situated in front
of the knee SYN: kneecap.
"The **patella** is a type of *sesamoid* bone
embedded within a tendon."
patellar (*adj.*)

patient-controlled analgesia (*abbrev.*)
\pɪ:-sɪ:-'eɪ\ a device that infuses
narcotics via an IV or epidural catheter
"A **PCA** pump lets the patient push
a button to administer pain meds as
needed."

PCA

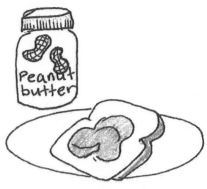

peanut butter
\'pɪ:-nʌt 'bʌ-dʒ:\ a food item made of
peanut paste
"**Peanut butter** and jelly is a popular
sandwich for children."

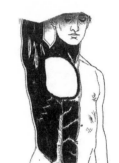

pectoral
\pek-'tɔ:-əl\ concerning the chest
"Resistance exercises like push-ups can
strengthen the **pectoral** muscles."

pediatric advanced life support
(*acronym*)
\pælz\ the protocols for treating medical
emergencies of infants and children
"**PALS** certification is required for those
who provide healthcare to children."

PALS

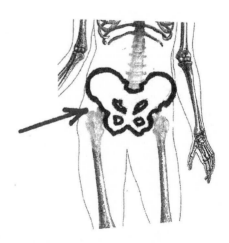

pelvis
\'pel-vɪs\ any basin-shaped structure
or cavity; the bony compartment of the
innominate bones, sacrum and coccyx
"The male **pelvis** and the female **pelvis**
differ in shape."

penicillin (*abbrev.*)
\pɪ:-sɪ:-'en\ a type of antibiotic
"Many types of bacteria are now
resistant to **PCN**."

PCN

percutaneous endoscopic gastrostomy
(*acronym*)
\peg\ a type of feeding tube
SYN: G-tube, gastrostomy.
"All meds given via **PEG** tube."

PEG

percutaneous endoscopic jejunostomy
(*acronym*)
\pedʒ\ a type of feeding tube
SYN: J-tube.
"He has a **PEJ** due to recurrent
aspiration pneumonia."

PEJ

percutaneous transluminal coronary
angioplasty (*abbrev.*)
\pɪ:-tɪ:-sɪ:-'eɪ\ an invasive vascular
procedure
"Some blocked coronary arteries can
be treated with **PTCA** instead of a
CABG."

PTCA

perineum
\peə-ə-'nɪ-əm\ the structures of the
pelvic outlet and the skin surrounding
the area
"A bedfast patient needs extra care in
keeping the **perineum** clean and dry to
prevent skin breakdown."

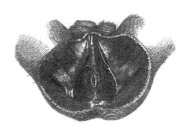

peripherally inserted central catheter
(*acronym*)
\pɪk\ a type of IV line that extends into
a large vein
"You can draw blood from the **PICC**
line."

PICC

per os
\pɪː-'əʊ\ Latin for "by mouth"
"He's not taking anything **p.o.** right now."

p.o.

personal protective equipment
(*abbrev.*)
\pɪː-pɪː-'ɪː\ protective clothing worn in the hospital
"**PPE** includes a gown, gloves, mask, and goggles."

PPE

pharynx
\'feə-ɪːnks\ the passageway for air from the nasal cavity to the larynx and for food from the mouth to the esophagus
SYN: throat.
"A Yankauer is used to clear secretions from the **oropharynx**."
pharyngeal (*adj.*)

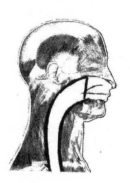

Abbreviation for **phencyclidine**
(*drug*); **primary care provider** (*title*);
pneumocystis carinii pneumonia
(*disease*)
\pɪː-sɪː-'pɪː\
"Follow up with your **PCP** in one week."

PCP

the symbol for **phosphate**
\pɪː-əʊ-'fɔː\ any salt of phosphoric acid containing the radical PO_4
"A low level of **phosphate** in the blood is called *hypophosphatemia*."

PO4

physical therapy (*abbrev.*)
\pɪː-'tɪː\ a department in the hospital
"The patient can start getting up with **PT** today."

P.T.

Physician's Desk Reference® (*abbrev.*)
\pɪ:-dɪ:-'ɑ:\ a book of drug listings
"You can look up pill information in the
PDR®."

piercing
\'pɪə-sɪ:ŋ\ a perforation of a body part
for decoration
"Check all **piercings** and remove any
jewelry before taking the patient to
MRI."
piercings (*pl.*)

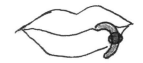

pig
\pɪg\ a wild or domestic swine
"'The Three Little **Pigs**' is a story that
many American children know."
pigs (*pl.*)

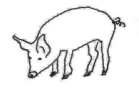

pill
\pɪl\ medicine in a small rounded mass
to be swallowed whole
"Here's your pain **pill**."

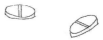

pill bottle
\pɪl 'bɒ-dəl\ a container for holding
tablets or capsules
"She has several **pill bottles** in her
purse."
bottles (*pl.*)

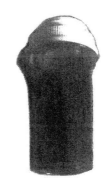

pillow
\'pɪ-ləʊ\ a cushion or pad to support the
head while reclining
"Would you like an extra **pillow** under
your head?"

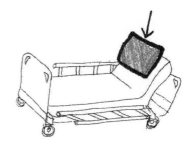

pinkie
\'pɪːn-kɪː\ the fifth and smallest finger
of the hand SYN: little finger.
"I'll put this pulse ox on your **pinkie**."

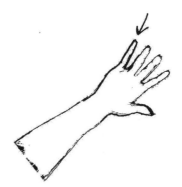

placenta
\plə-'sen-tə\ a structure in the uterus
that provides oxygen and nourishment
to the fetus
"Another name for the expelled
placenta is *afterbirth*."

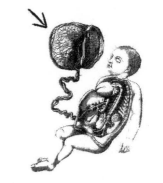

place setting
\pleɪs 'se-dɪːŋ\ a table service for one
person
"A **place setting** usually consists of
dishes, silverware, and a napkin."

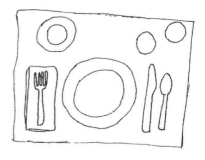

plaid
\plæd\ a pattern of unevenly spaced repeated stripes crossing at right angles
"His clothing includes one **plaid** flannel shirt."

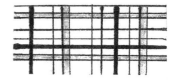

plate
\pleɪt\ a shallow usually circular dish to hold food
"I can't eat this whole **plate** of food."

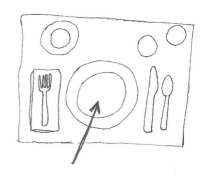

platelets (*abbrev.*)
\'pleɪt-ləts\ a blood component
"**Plts.** are thrombocytes that contribute to blood clotting."

plts

point
\pɔɪnt\ to indicate the position of direction; a small mark; the purpose of something
"**Point** to where it hurts."

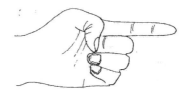

point-of-care testing (*abbrev.*)
\pɔɪnt-ʌv-keə-'tes-tɪːŋ\ medical testing at or near the site of patient care
"**POCT** is completed at the bedside."

POCT

polka dots
\'pəʊ-kə dɒts\ a pattern of regularly distributed dots
"I lost my umbrella; it is black with white **polka dots.**"

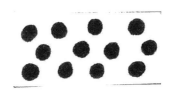

pollex
\'pɒ-ləks\ the first finger of the hand
SYN: thumb.
"The word *thumb* is much more
commonly used than *pollex*."

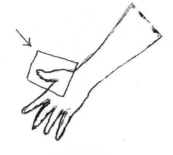

ponytail
\'pəʊ-nɪ:-teɪl\ a hairstyle with the hair
banded together in the back of the head
"Let's put your hair in a **ponytail** to
keep it out of the way."

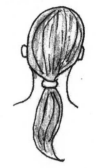

pork
\pɔ:k\ the meat of the pig
"Ham and bacon are **pork** products."

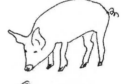

positron emission tomography
(acronym)
\pet\ a type of nuclear medicine scan
"A **PET** scan is one diagnostic tool for
cancer."

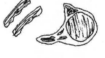

PET

positive end-expiratory pressure
(acronym)
\pɪ:p\ a ventilator setting
"The patient is on the ventilator with a
PEEP of 10."

PEEP

positive symbol
\'pɒ-zɪ-tɪv\ definite, affirmative; real
and numerically greater than zero
"That patient with diarrhea is C. diff +."

post-anesthesia care unit (*abbrev.*)
\pɪ-eɪ-sɪ:-'juː\ a department in the
hospital
"Patients are transferred to the **PACU**
after surgery to recover."

PACU

post merideum
\'pɪ:-em\ Latin for "evening"; the time
period from twelve to midnight
"Dinner should be here around 6:00
p.m."

p.m.

post-traumatic stress disorder
(*abbrev.*)
\pɪ:-tɪ:-es-'dɪ:\ a group of psychiatric
symptoms
"Many soldiers who have been in
combat have **PTSD**."

PTSD

pot
\pɒt\ marijuana SYN: weed.
"A toxicology screen lists **pot** as
cannabinoids."

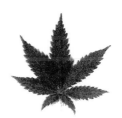

the symbol for the element **potassium**
\pə-'tæ-sɪ:-əm\ an electrolyte
"Check a **K+** level after each KCl bolus
given."

K+

the formula for **potassium chloride**
\keɪ-sɪ:-'el\ two electrolytes in the body
"The patient's IV is D5 1/2NS with 20
mEq **KCl** @ 100 cc/hr."

KCl

the formula for **potassium hydroxide**
\keɪ-əʊ-'eɪʧ\ a chemical solution used
in the laboratory
"Some lab tests include a **KOH** slide."

KOH

the formula for **potassium phosphate**
\'keɪ-fɒs\ a chemical solution to
replenish blood levels
"Add some **KPO**$_4$ to the next bag of IV
fluids please."

KPO4

potty chair
\'pɒ-dɪ: ʧeə\ a small portable toilet
SYN: BSC, commode.
"Could you bring that **potty chair** over
here for me, please?"

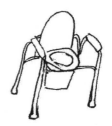

the symbol for **pound**
\paʊnd\ a unit of weight
"1 **lb.** equals sixteen ounces."

lb.

povidone-iodine
\'pəʊ-vɪ-dəʊn-'aɪ-əʊ-daɪn\ a
solution used as a surgical scrub and
antibacterial agent
"A commonly used brand name for
povidone-iodine is *Betadine*®
\'beɪ-də-daɪn\."

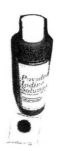

premature ventricular contraction
(*abbrev.*)
\pɪːvɪ-'sɪː\ a type of wave on the EKG
reading
"A **PVC** is a type of ventricular ectopy."

PVC

prescription (*abbrev.*)
\prə-'skrɪp-ʃən\ a written direction or order for dispensing and administering drugs
"**Rx**: take one tablet TID with meals."

Rx

P-R interval
\pɪ-'ɑː\ portion of the EKG from the beginning of the P-wave to the beginning of the QRS complex; atrial depolarization
"A normal **P-R** interval is < 0.20 sec."

P-R

private branch exchange system (*abbrev.*)
\pɪ:-bɪ:-'eks\ a telephone system
"**PBX** is another name for the hospital telephone operator."

PBX

prone
\prəʊn\ horizontal with the face downward
"The **prone** position is discouraged for newborns due to the risk of SIDS."

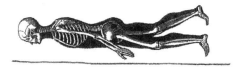

pro re nata
\pɪ:-ɑ:-'en\ Latin for "as necessary"
"Morphine is ordered **prn** pain."

prn

prostatic specific antigen (*abbrev.*)
\pɪ:-es-'eɪ\ a cancer marker
"Men with an enlarged prostate gland should have their **PSA** level checked."

PSA

prosthesis
\prɒs-'θɪ:-sɪs\ an artifical substitute for a missing body part
"The amputee walks with a **prosthetic** leg."
prosthetic (*adj.*)

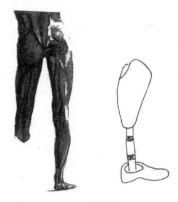

proximal
\'prɒk-sə-məl\ toward or nearest the center of the body
"The **proximal** tibia forms part of the knee joint."

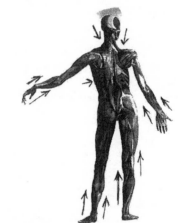

pudding
\'pʊ-dɪːŋ\ a soft, creamy dessert food
"We have some tapioca **pudding** for a snack."

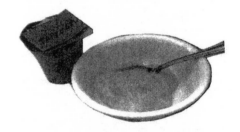

pupils equal and reactive to light
(*acronym*)
\pɜːl\ a description of pupil response
"Alert, **PERL**, face symmetric, grips equal."

PERL

pulmonary function tests (*abbrev.*)
\pɪ:-ef-'tɪ:z\ a test to measure lung
volumes
"**PFTs** can measure lung capacity."

PFT's

pulseless electrical activity (*abbrev.*)
\pɪ:-ɪ:-'eɪ\ a condition of cardiac arrest
that produces an EKG waveform but no
pulse
"During the code, the patient was found
to be in **PEA**."

PEA

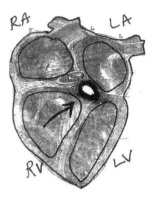

pulmonic valve
\pʌl-'mɒ-nɪk vælv\ the heart valve
between the right ventricle and the
pulmonary artery
"Blood passes through the **pulmonic
valve** on its way to the lungs."

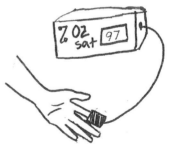

pulse ox
\'pʌls ɒks\ a measure of oxygen
saturation SYN: SpO$_2$, oximetry.
"A **pulse ox** probe can be placed on the
ear lobe as well as a finger."

pupils
\'pju:-pəlz\ the black opening in the
center of the eyes
"Normal **pupils** are equal and reactive
to light."

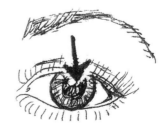

purified protein derivative (*abbrev.*)
\pɪ:-pɪ:-'dɪ:\ a testing agent
"A **PPD** is a TB skin test."

P.P.D.

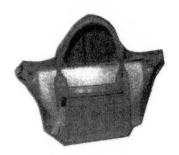

purse
\pɜ:s\ a bag to carry personal belongings
and money
"The patient chose to keep her **purse** at
the bedside."

Chapter Seventeen

Qq \kju:\
The letter *Q* is the seventeenth letter of the English alphabet.

Q is for *queen*. \kwɪːn\
"In chess, the **queen** is always on her color."

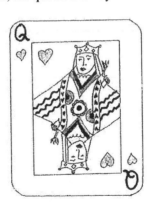

Q

\kju:\ indicates *each* or *every*
"Please weigh the patient **Q** day."

Q

QHS

\kju:-eɪʧ-'es\ every night at bedtime
"MOM 30 ml **QHS** prn constipation."

QHS

every other day (*abbrev.*)

\kju:-'əʊ-dɪ:\ a designation of frequency
"Her Coumadin schedule right now is
only 1 mg **QOD**."

QOD

QRS

\kju:-ɑ:-'es\ the portion of an EKG
waveform representing ventricular
depolarization
"A PVC may look like a wide and
bizarre **QRS**."

QRS

\kju:-ɑ:-'es\ the pattern on the EKG
that represents depolarization of the
ventricles
"The heart rate can usually be measured
by counting the **QRS** complexes."

QRS

Q-T

\kju:-'tɪ:\ the representation on the
EKG of ventricular depolarization and
repolarization
"A lengthening **Q-T** interval can lead to
ventricular dysrhythmias."

Q-T

QTc
\kju:-tɪ:-'sɪ:\ the duration of the Q-T
interval adjusted for the patient's heart
rate
"A **QTc** is monitored when giving IV
haloperidol."

QTc

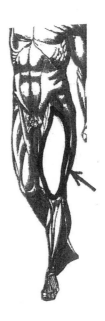

quadriceps
\'kwɒ-drɪ-seps\ the large muscle on the
anterior surface of the thigh
"Lunges with weights can help to
strengthen the **quadriceps** muscles."

quantity sufficient (*abbrev.*)
\kju:-'es\ an adequate amount
"UO **QS** via catheter."

QS

quaque die
\kju:-'dɪ:\ Latin for "once a day"
"He takes one baby aspirin **QD**."

QD

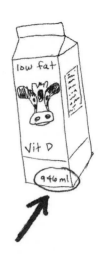

quart
\kwɔ:t\ a unit of fluid equal to one
fourth of a gallon
"One **quart** is thirty-two ounces."

quater in die
\kju:-ɑɪ-'dɪ:\ Latin for "four times a
day"
"The surgeon would like him to get up
and walk **QID**."

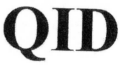

quotation marks
\kwəʊ-'teɪ-ʃən mɑ:ks\ a pair of
punctuation marks to indicate the
beginning and the end of a quotation
Example: The patient said he "feels like
crap" this morning.

Chapter Eighteen

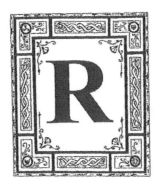

Rr \ɑ:\
The letter *R* is the eighteenth letter of the English alphabet.

R is for *rabbit*. \'ræ-bət\
"Bugs Bunny is a famous American **rabbit**."

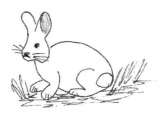

radiation
\reɪ-dɪ:-'eɪ-ʃən\ a caution symbol
"The CT scanner will have a **radiation** symbol displayed."

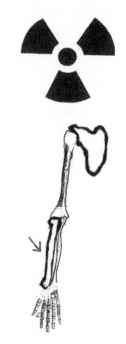

radius
\'reɪ-dɪ:-əs\ one of the forearm bones on the thumb side
"The **radius** is the shorter bone of the forearm."
radial (*adj.*)

rapid ventricular response (*abbrev.*)
\ɑ:-vɪ:-'ɑ:\ a cardiac rhythm analysis
"Admission diagnosis is AF with **RVR**."

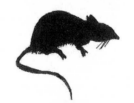

rat
\ræt\ rodent, genus *Rattus*
"**Rats** can spread bubonic plague."
rats (*pl.*)

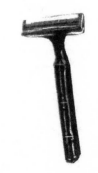

razor
\'reɪ-zɜ:\ a sharp metal cutting instrument used for shaving
"Disposable safety **razors** or electric trimmers are used in the hospital to remove hair."

razor blade
\'reɪ-zɜ: bleɪd\ the sharp piece of metal inside a razor
"A scalpel and a **razor blade** are both dangerously sharp instruments."

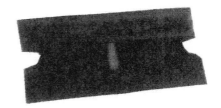

receiving blanket
\rə-'sɪ:-vɪ:ŋ 'blæn-kət\ a flannel blanket for swaddling babies
"Infants are wrapped in a **receiving blanket** for warmth and security."

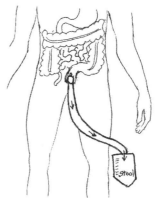

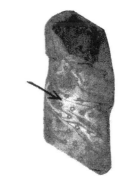

rectal tube
\'rek-təl tu:b\ a soft flexible tube for draining stool from the rectum
"The patient with diarrhea has a **rectal tube** in place."

rectangle
\'rek-tæŋ-əl\ a parallelogram all of whose angles are right angles
"A hospital pillow is **rectangular** in shape."
rectangular (*adj.*)

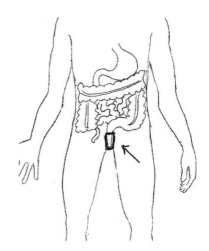

rectum
\'rek-təm\ the final portion of the large intestine
"A fecal impaction was noted in the **rectum** on x-ray."

red blood cells (*abbrev.*)
\ɑ:-bɪ:-'sɪ:z\ one component of blood
"A high **RBC** count is called *polycythemia*."

RBC

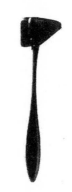

reflex hammer
\'rɪ:-fleks 'hæ-mɜ:\ a small rubber mallet used to check nerve responses
"An otoscope and **reflex hammer** are in the doctor's examination tray."

registered nurse (*abbrev.*)
\ɑ:-'en\ a title
"The charge nurse is an **RN**."

RN

regulator
\'reg-ju:-leɪ-dɜː\ a valve for an oxygen
outlet
"You can't use an oxygen tank without a
regulator."

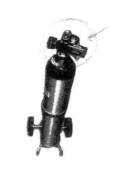

respirator
\'res-pɜː-eɪ-dɜː\ a machine used to assist
ventilation and oxygenation
SYN: life support, ventilator.
"He is still recovering on an artificial
respirator."

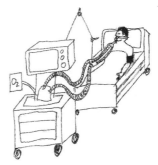

respiratory rate (*abbrev.*)
\'res-pɪ-tɔː-rɪː reɪt\ how fast a patient is
breathing
"The patient is tachypneic with a **RR** of
40."

RR

respiratory therapist (*title*);
respiratory therapy (*abbrev.*)
\ɑː-'tɪː\
"Would you please call **RT** for a
breathing treatment?"

R.T.

retina
\'re-tə-nə\ the innermost layer of the
eye that contains the receptors for
vision
"One complication of diabetes is
damage to the **retina**, which is called
retinopathy."

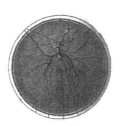

return of spontaneous circulation
(abbrev.)
\ɑ:-əʊ-es-'sɪ:\ a resumption of
sustained perfusing heart activity after a
cardiopulmonary arrest
"**ROSC** is the goal of CPR."

ROSC

review of systems
\rɪ:-'vju: ʌv 'sɪs-təmz\ a doctor's
description of a physical examination
"**ROS** is part of the doctor's H&P."

ROS

ribs
\rɪbz\ the bones of the thorax that encase
the lungs
"Broken **ribs** are very painful because it
hurts to breathe."

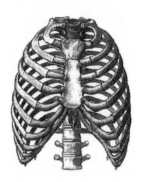

right angle
\rɑɪt 'æŋ-əl\ a ninety-degree angle
"In high Fowler's position, the patient is
sitting up at a **right angle**."

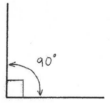

right coronary artery *(abbrev.)*
\ɑ:-sɪ:-'eɪ\ an artery that supplies blood
to both ventricles
"The patient had an **RCA** stenting done
six months ago."

RCA

ring
\rɪːŋ\ a piece of jewelry worn on the finger
"The patient's **ring** was removed because his hands were swollen."

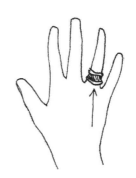

ring finger
\rɪːŋ 'fɪːŋ-ɜːˌ\ the fourth finger of the hand
"He fell and broke his right **ring finger**."

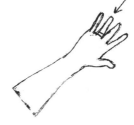

robe
\rəʊb\ a loose garment for informal wear
"I'd like to put on my **robe** and take a walk."

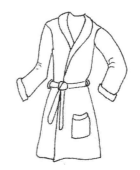

rotator cuff
\'rəʊ-teɪ-dɜː kʌf\ a group of four tendons that attach to the shoulder joint capsule
"I had a **rotator cuff** repair done last year."

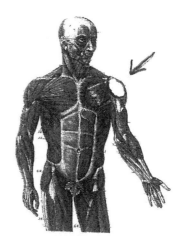

rubber band
\rʌ-bɜ:-'bænd\ a continous small band
of rubber used to hold things together
"Do you have a **rubber band** so I can
put my hair in a ponytail?"

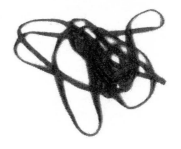

ruler
\'ru:-lɜ:\ a hard measuring stick
"A measuring tape is like a soft, flexible
ruler."

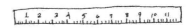

Chapter Nineteen

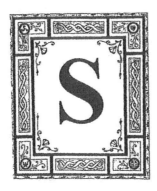

Ss \es\
The letter *S* is the nineteenth letter of the English alphabet.

S is for *star*. \stɑ:\
"American children recite the alphabet to the tune of 'Twinkle, Twinkle Little **Star**.'"

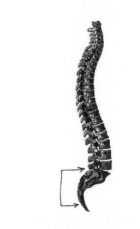

sacrum

\'seɪ-krəm\ the triangular bone between
the fifth lumber vertebra and the spine
"The male and female **sacrum** differ in
shape."
sacral (*adj.*)

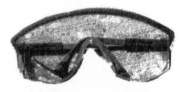

safety goggles

\'seɪf-tɪ: 'gɒ-gəlz\ plastic glasses worn
to protect the eyes
"**Safety goggles** are part of personal
protective equipment."

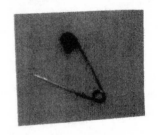

safety pin

\'seɪf-tɪ: pɪn\ a pin in the form of a clasp
with a guard covering its point when
fastened
"A **safety pin** can be used to check a
patient's perception of sharpness or
dullness."

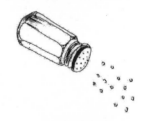

salt

\sɒlt\ a crystalline compound of NaCl
used to season food
"Too much **salt** is bad for your
congestive heart failure."

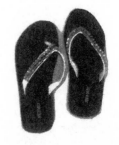

sandals

\'sæn-dəlz\ lighter shoes consisting of
soles strapped to the feet
"I was only wearing **sandals** when I
injured my foot."

saturation of peripheral oxygen
(*abbrev.*)
\es-pɪ:-əʊ-'tu:\ a measure of a patient's oxygenation status SYN: pulse ox.
"Keep SpO_2 89-92% for the COPD patient."

SpO2

Saturday (*abbrev.*)
\'sæ-dɜ:-deɪ\ the seventh day of the week
"Public schools are usually closed on **Sat.**"

Sat.

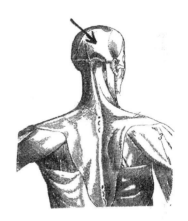

scalp
\skælp\ the skin that covers the skull
"**Scalp** lacerations can bleed quite a bit."

scalpel
\'skæl-pəl\ a very sharp blade used for cutting in surgery
"**Scalpel** blades are disposed of in the sharps container."

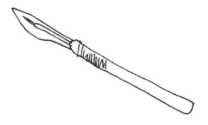

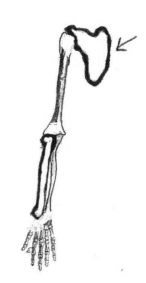

scapula
\'skæp- juː-lə\ the large flat triangular
bone that forms the posterior part of the
shoulder SYN: shoulder blade.
"The patient complains of pain radiating
to the mid**scapular** area."
scapular (*adj.*)

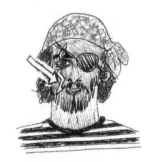

scar
\skɑː\ a mark left on the skin by the
healing of a wound
"The surgical **scar** is fully healed."

scissors
\'sɪ-zɜːz\ a cutting instrument with two
blades whose cutting edges slide past
each other
"Would you please get me some sterile
scissors for this dressing change?"

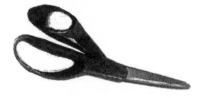

scoliosis

\skəʊ-lɪː-'əʊ-səs\ a lateral curvature of the spine

"The patient has chronic low back pain from **scoliosis**."

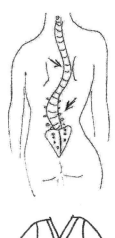

scrubs

\skrʌbz\ sterile clothing worn by OR personnel; also hospital uniforms

"The hospital would like the nurses to all wear the same color **scrubs**."

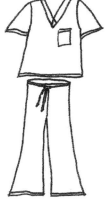

second

\'se-kənd\ an ordinal number indicating number 2 in a series

"Attempt a **2nd** dose of adenosine if the first one has no effect."

2nd

September (*abbrev.*)

\sep-'tem-bɜː\ the ninth month of the year

"Labor Day is on the first Monday in **Sept**."

Sept.

sequential compression devices
\e-sɪ:-'dɪːz\ pumps placed on the legs to promote circulation
"VTE prophylaxis includes applying **sequential compression devices**."

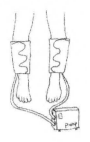

sequential compression devices
(*abbrev.*)
\e-sɪ:-'dɪːz\
"**SCDs** are placed on surgical patients."

SCD's

seventh
\'se-vənθ\ an ordinal number indicating number 7 in a series
"Pearl Harbor Day is December **7th**."

7th

sexually transmitted disease (*abbrev.*)
\es-tɪ:-'dɪː\ a group of diseases that can be spread by sexual contact, such as gonorrhea
"Another name for **STD** is *venereal disease*."

STD

sharps container
\ʃɑːps kən-'teɪ-nɜ:\ a disposal bin for used medical needles and other sharp objects
"Glass vials should be thrown away in the **sharps container**."

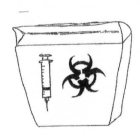

shellfish
\'ʃel-fɪʃ\ an aquatic invertebrate animal
with a shell
"Some religious dietary laws forbid the
eating of **shellfish**."

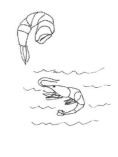
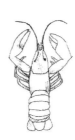

shin
\ʃɪnz\ the anterior edge of the tibia.
"Soccer players wear **shin** guards to
protect their legs."

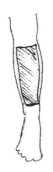
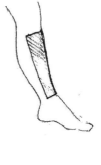

shirt
\ʃɜ:t\ a garment for the upper part of the
body
"That doctor always wears a **shirt** and
tie to work."

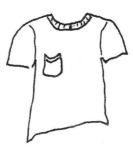

shoes
\ʃu:z\ outer coverings for the human foot
"OSHA has safety standards for **shoes**
in the workplace."

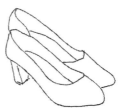

short of breath (*abbrev.*)
\ʃɔ:t ʌv 'briːθ\ difficulty breathing;
dyspneic
"The patient is very **SOB** with any
exertion."

shorts
\ʃɔ:ts\ knee-length or less than
knee-length pants
"It's so hot today I should have worn
shorts."

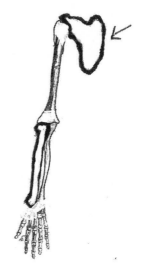

shoulder blade
\'ʃʌl-dʒ: bleɪd\ the large flat triangular
bone that forms the posterior part of the
shoulder SYN: scapula.
"The acromion process is a point on the
shoulder blade."

shoulders
\'ʃʌl-dʒ:z\ the region at the top of each
arm where the proximal humerus,
clavicle, and scapula connect
"Muscle tension in the **shoulders** and
neck can cause headaches."

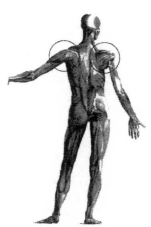

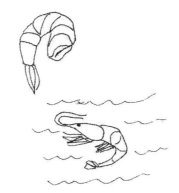

shrimp

\ʃrɪmp\ a small marine decapod crustacean that is a popular food
"A patient allergic to **shrimp** may also have an iodine allergy."

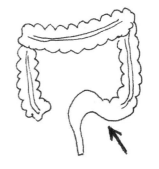

siderails

\'sɑɪd-reɪlz\ bars on the sides of a bed or gurney to prevent patient falls
"Keep the **siderails** up while the patient is sleeping."

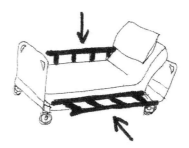

sigmoid colon

\'sɪg-mɔɪd 'kəʊ-lən\ the S-shaped final portion of the colon
"A *sigmoidoscopy* is an examination of the **sigmoid colon**."

silverware
\'sɪl-vɜ:-weə\ a name for eating utensils
"We use plastic, disposable **silverware**
in the cafeteria."

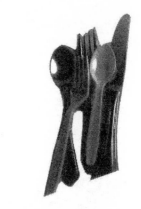

sink
\sɪ:nk\ a stationary basin connected to a
drain and water supply for washing and
draining
"Many **sinks** in the hospital have
faucets controlled by foot pedals."
sinks (*pl.*)

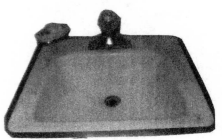

sinus bradycardia (*abbrev.*)
\'saɪ-nəs breɪ-dɪ-'ka:-dɪ:-ə\ a slow
heart rhythm
"**SB** is SR with a rate less than 60 bpm."

SB

sinus rhythm (*abbrev.*)
\'saɪ-nəs 'rɪ-θəm\ a normal heart
rhythm
"The patient converted to **SR** after
initial amiodarone infusion."

SR

sinus tachycardia (*abbrev.*)
\'saɪ-nəs tæk\ a fast heart rhythm
"A child with an elevated temperature
may have **ST**."

ST

sixth
\sɪksə\ an ordinal number indicating
number 6 in a series
"Intuition is sometimes called a **6th**
sense."

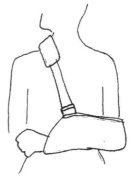

skeleton
\'ske-lə-tən\ the bones of the body
"The human **skeleton** is made up of 206
bones."

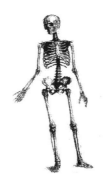

skull
\skʌl\ the bony framework of the head
SYN: cranium.
"A **skull** and crossbones is a symbol of
poison or danger to life."

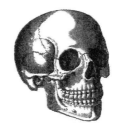

sling
\slɪːŋ\ a support for an injured upper
extremity
"Keep your arm elevated and in this
sling while it is healing."

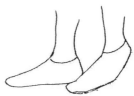

slippers
\'slɪ-pɜːz\ a light shoe that is easily
slipped onto the foot
"I have some bedroom **slippers** in the
closet."

smile
\smaɪl\ a facial expression in which
the eyes brighten and the corners of the
mouth curve slightly upward
"Asking the patient to **smile** is part of a
neurological assessment."

smiley face
\'smaɪ-lɪ: feɪs\ a cartoon image of a
smiling face SYN: happy face.
"A **smiley face** is often used to convey
happiness or appreciation."

snake
\sneɪk\ a limbless scaled reptile with a
long tapering body
"**Snake** venom can contain neurotoxins
or hemotoxins."

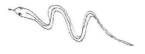

socks
\sɒks\ a knitted or woven covering for
the foot
"Please put some **socks** on when you
get OOB."

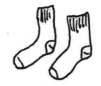

the symbol for the **sodium ion**
\'səʊ-dɪ:-əm\ an electrolyte
"A low serum **Na+** is called
hyponatremia."

Na+

the formula for **sodium chloride**
\'səʊ-dɪ:-əm 'klɔ:-aɪd\ salt
"*Normal saline* is 0.9% **NaCl**."

NaCl

specimen cup
\'spe-sə-mən kʌp\ a plastic container to
hold laboratory samples
"Make sure you tighten the lid of the
specimen cup so the contents don't
spill."

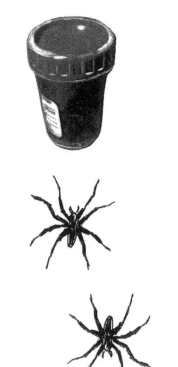

spider
\'spɑɪ-dɝ:\ a crawling insect (arachnid)
that can spin a web and may have a
poisonous bite
"The brown recluse **spider** is
poisonous."

spider bite
\'spɑɪ-dɝ: bɑɪt\ the injury caused by the
bite of a poisonous spider
"A black widow **spider bite** can cause
muscle cramps, nausea, and vomiting."

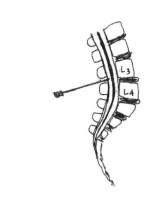

spinal tap
\'spɑɪ-nəl tæp\ the process of entering
the subarachnoid space to obtain
cerebrospinal fluid SYN: lumbar
puncture.
"Have the patient sign a consent form
for the **spinal tap**."

spine
\spɑɪn\ the spinal column; the bones of
the back SYN: the backbone.
"**Spinal** stenosis causes a narrowing of
the **spinal** canal."
spinal (*adj.*)

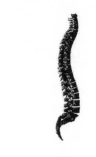

spit pan
\spɪt pæn\ a receptacle for
expectorating or vomiting SYN: emesis
basin.
"I feel sick; I need that **spit pan**."

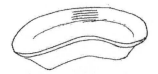

spleen
\splɪ:n\ a lymphoid organ in the upper
left abdominal quadrant
"The **spleen** may be removed for a
condition such as ITP."

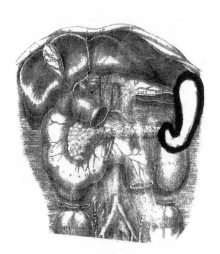

spoon
\spu:n\ an eating or cooking utensil
shaped like a small bowl with a handle
"His hands are too weak to hold a **spoon**
so he needs help to eat."

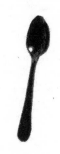

square
\skweə\ a figure with four equal sides
and four right angles
"2 × 2s and 4 × 4s are **square**
dressings."

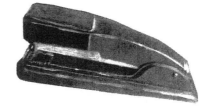

stapler
\'steɪp-lɜː\ a small device for inserting
wire staples
"There should be a **stapler** at the desk."

staples
\'steɪ-pəlz\ articles for fastening tissues
together during surgery
"The surgeon asked me to remove every
other **staple** from your incision."
staple (*s.*)

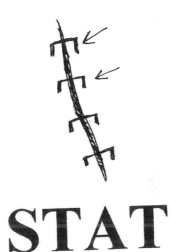

statim (*acronym*)
\stæt\ Latin for "immediately"
"We need an ABG **STAT** please."

STAT

S-T elevation
\'es-tɪ el-ə-'veɪ-ʃən\ a sign on the EKG
that may indicate myocardial ischemia
"The patient with **S-T elevation** was
transferred to the cardiac cath lab for
immediate intervention."

sterile towel
\'steə-əl 'tɑʊ-əl\ a towel that has been
autoclaved
"A **sterile towel** is used to create a
sterile field."

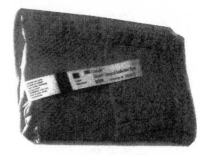

sternum
\'stɜ:-nəm\ the narrow, flat bone in the
middle of the thorax
SYN: breastbone.
"The patient has **sternal** wires in place
from a prior CABG."
sternal (*adj.*)

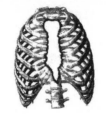

stethoscope
\'steə-ə-skəʊp\ an instrument used to
transmit sounds from the body to the
examiner's ears
"A **stethoscope** is used for
auscultation."

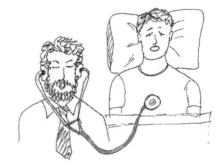

stomach
\'stʌ-mək\ a muscular, distensible
saclike portion of the alimentary
tube between the esophagus and the
duodenum SYN: belly.
"A gastric banding procedure reduces
the size of the **stomach**."

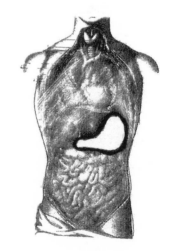

stool
\stu:l\ a seat usually without a back or
arms; the products of the colon
"The doctor sits on a low **stool** to help
deliver a baby."

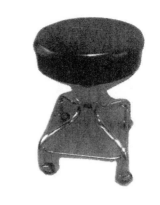

straighten
\'streɪ-ʔən\ to stretch out
"**Straighten** your right leg, please."

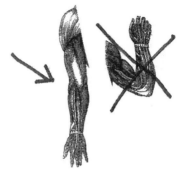

straw
\strɒ\ a tube for sucking up a beverage
"Do you prefer to swallow your pills
with or without a **straw**?"

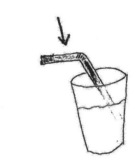

striped
\strɑɪpt\ having a pattern of lines that
vary in color
"A candy cane is **striped**."
stripe (*n.*)

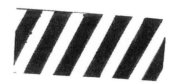

subcutaneous (*abbrev.*)
\sʌb-'kju:\ a route for an injection
"Taking narcotics by **SQ** injection is
called *skin popping*."

SQ

sublingual (*abbrev.*)
\sʌb-'lɪ:ŋ-wəl\ under the tongue
"NTG can be given **SL**."

SL

suction (*abbrev.*)
\'sʌk-ʃən\ the drawing of fluids using
negative pressure
"We need a continuous **sx** set up for this
procedure."

Sx

suitcase
\'su:t-keɪs\ a bag or case carried by hand
designed to hold a traveler's clothing
and personal items
"All my stuff is in my **suitcase**."

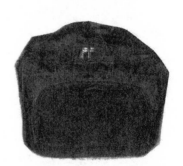

the symbol for **sulfate**
\'sʌl-feɪt\ a salt or ester of sulfuric acid
"Another name for $FeSO_4$ is *iron*."

SO4

Sunday (*abbrev.*)
\'sʌn-deɪ\ the first day of the week
"Many people attend church on **Sun**."

Sun.

supine
\'su:-paɪn\ lying on the back with the
face upward
"The patient is lying **supine** with the
HOB elevated."

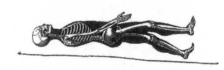

suppository
\sʌ-'pɒ-zɪ-tɔ:-ɪ:\ a semisolid substance containing medicine for introduction into the rectum, where it dissolves
"An obtunded pt. with a high fever needs an acetaminophen **suppository**."

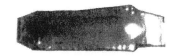
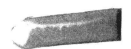

Surgical Care Improvement Project
(*abbrev.*)
\e-sɪ:-ɑɪ-'pɪ:\ a plan to reduce surgical complications
"VTE prophylaxis is one element of the **SCIP**."

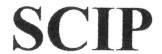

sutures
\'su:-ʧ3:z\ the thread, wire, or other material used to stitch parts of the body together
"Some **sutures** are designed to be absorbed by the body."

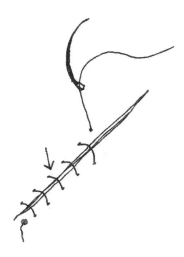

swab
\swɒb\ cotton or gauze at the end of a slender stick
SYN: cotton-tipped applicator
"Pack the wound gently using a **swab**."

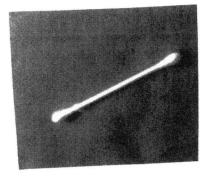

sweater
\'swe-dɜː\ a knitted or crocheted jacket
or pullover
"Can I wear my **sweater** to keep my
arms warm?"

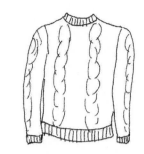

syringe
\sə-'rɪnʤ\ a cylindrical device used to
inject or withdraw fluids
"A tuberculin **syringe** usually holds 1 ml."

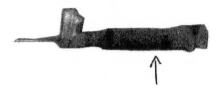

systemic lupus erythrematosus
(*abbrev.*)
\es-el-'ɪː\ an autoimmune disease
"**SLE** patients may have a butterfly rash
on the face."

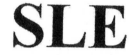

Chapter Twenty

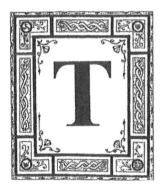

Tt \tɪ:\
The letter *T* is the twentieth letter of the English alphabet.

T is for *train.* \treɪn\
"Another word for **train** is *locomotive.*"

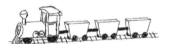

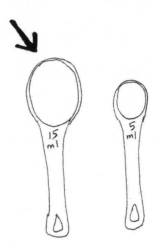

tablespoon
\'teɪ-bəl-spuːn\ a unit of measure used
in cooking
"One **tablespoon** equals 15 ml."

tablespoon (*abbrev.*)
\'teɪ-bəl-spuːn\ a unit of measure
"Take 1 **T** mixed in 8 oz. of water Q
day."

tablet
\'tæb-lət\ a small mass of medication to
be swallowed
"Do you want the KCl in **tablet** or
liquid form?"

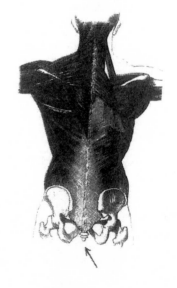

tailbone
\'teɪl-bəʊn\ the small bone at the base
of the spinal column SYN: coccyx.
"She slipped on ice and broke her
tailbone."

tampon
\'tæm-pɒn\ a small pack of absorbent
material used to collect menstrual blood
in the vagina
"*Toxic shock syndrome* is one possible
complication of leaving a **tampon** in
too long."

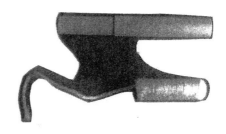

tape
\teɪp\ a narrow strip of material with
adhesive on one side
"Paper **tape** is better for sensitive skin."

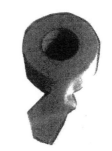

tarsus
\'tɑ:-səs\ the bones of the ankle
"The malleolus connects with the
tarsus."
tarsal (*adj.*)

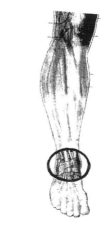

tattoo
\tæ-'tu:\ an indelible mark made on the
skin with pigment
"Many young people have **tattoos**."
tattoos (*pl.*)

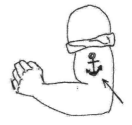

tea
\tɪː\ a beverage prepared with tea leaves
soaked in boiling water
"I would like **tea** instead of coffee,
please."

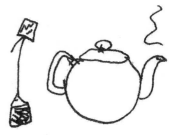

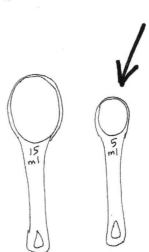

teaspoon
\'tɪː-spuːn\ a small spoon that is used for
stirring beverages and also as a measure
in cooking
"One **teaspoon** equals 5 ml."

teaspoon (*abbrev.*)
\'tɪː-spuːn\ a small spoon that is used for
stirring beverages and also as a measure
in cooking
"Take 2 **t.** every 4 hours prn cough."

t.

teeth
\tɪːθ\ the small bones in the jaw used for
chewing
SYN: dentition.
"Can I help you brush your **teeth**?"

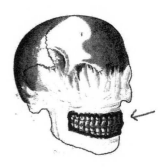

telephone
\'te-lə-fəʊn\ an instrument of
communication that transmits sounds
by wire
"Just dial 9 to get an outside **telephone**
line."

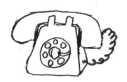

television (*abbrev.*)
\'tɪ:-vɪ:\ an electronic system of
transmitting images and sound
"Would you like to watch **TV**?"

T.V.

temporal lobe
\'tem-pɜ:-əl ləʊb\ the lobes of the
cerebrum lying on the sides of the head
above the ears
"One of the left **temporal lobe**
functions is the processing of language."

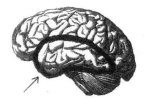

temperature (*abbrev.*)
\temp\ the degree of hotness or coldness
of a substance
"Draw blood cultures prn **temp** >
101.5."

temp

tenth
\tenθ\ an ordinal number indicating
number 10 in a series
"October is the **10th** month of the year."

10th

ter in die
\tɪ:-ɑɪ-'dɪ:\ Latin for "three times a day"
"**TID** may be the same frequency as
Q8h."

TID

testicles
\'tes-tɪ-kəlz\ the male reproductive
glands that are located in the scrotum
SYN: gonads.
"The **testicles** produce testosterone and
spermatozoa."
testicular (*adj.*)

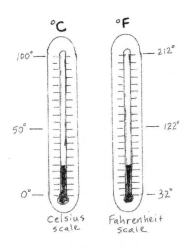

tetraiodothyronine (*abbrev.*)
\tɪ:-'fɔ:\ a thyroid hormone
SYN: thyroxine.
"A **T4** level is included in a thyroid
panel."

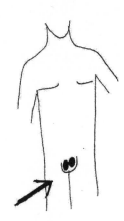

thermometer
\ɵ3:-'mɒ-mə-dɜ:\ an instrument for
determining temperature
"A urinary catheter **thermometer**
monitors core temperature."

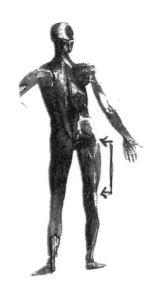

thigh
\θɑɪ\ the upper portion of the leg
"The **thigh** is one location for a subcutaneous insulin injection."

third
\θɜ:d\ an ordinal number indicating number 3 in a series
"The **3rd** time's the charm."

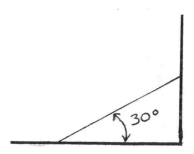

3rd

30 degrees
\'θɜ:-dɪ: də-'grɪ:z\ an angle or level of elevation that is often indicated for patients in hospital beds
"Keep HOB elevated **30 degrees** to prevent aspiration."

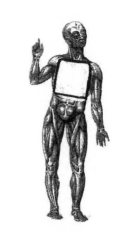

thorax
\'ɵɔ:-aks\ the portion of the body that
houses the chest cavity
"Emphysema can cause a barrel-shaped
thorax."

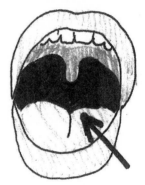

throat
\ɵrəʊt\ the inside of the neck from the
mouth and nose to the esophagus
"A streptococcal infection can cause a
sore **throat**."

thumb
\ɵʌm\ the first finger of the hand SYN:
pollex.
"In American culture, a **thumbs**-up sign
means all is well."
thumbs (*pl.*)

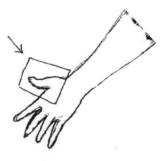

Thursday (*abbrev.*)
\'ɵɜ:z-deɪ\ the fifth day of the week
"Thanksgiving always falls on a **Thu**."

Thu.

thymus gland
\'θɑɪ-məs glænd\ a lymphoid organ located in the middle anterior chest
"The **thymus gland** is involved in T-cell production."

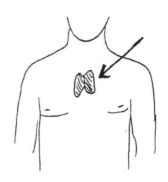

thyroid
\'θɑɪ-rɔɪd\ an endocrine gland that regulates metabolism
"An enlarged **thyroid** gland may be called a *goiter*."

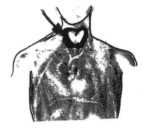

thyroid stimulating hormone (*abbrev.*)
\ti:-es-'eɪtʃ\ a hormone secreted by the pituitary
"A low **TSH** level may indicate a hyperactive thyroid gland."

TSH

tibia
\'tɪ-bɪ:-ə\ the larger bone of the lower leg
"The patient has a **tibial** plateau fracture."
tibial (*adj.*)

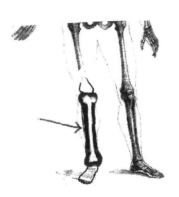

tissue plasminogen activator (*abbrev.*)
\tɪ:-pɪ:-'eɪ\ an enzyme that helps degrade blood clots
"The patient's blood clot was dissolved with **tPA**."

tPA

tissues
\'tɪ-ʃu:z\ soft absorbent papers used for
blotting nasal secretions
"A commonly used brand name for
tissues is *Kleenex®*
\'klɪ:-neks\."

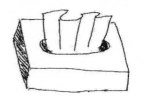

trimethoprim-sulfamethoxazole
(abbrev.)
\traɪ-'meθ-ə-prɪm sʌl-fə\ an antibiotic
drug
"**TMP-SMX** may be used to treat
urinary tract infections."

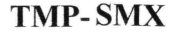

toenail
\'təʊ-neɪlz\ the hard portion of the
epidermis at the end of the toe
"That ingrown **toenail** is causing me
pain."

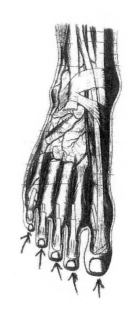

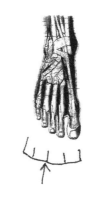

toes
\ˈtəʊz\ the digits of the feet
"Can you wiggle your **toes**, please?"

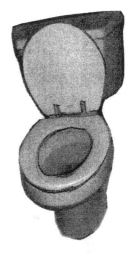

toilet
\ˈtɔɪ-lət\ a fixture designed for
defecation and urination
"**Toilets** are usually made of porcelain."
toilets (*pl.*)

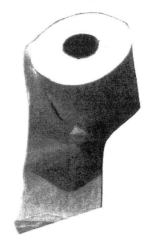

toilet paper
\ˈtɔɪ-let ˈpeɪ-pɜː\ thin paper used for
cleaning after using the toilet
"Can I have a new roll of **toilet paper**,
please?"

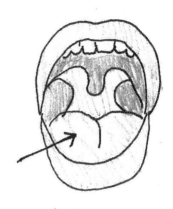

tongue
\tʌŋ\ the organ in the floor of the mouth
used for speech, taste, and swallowing
"Candida infections can cause a coated
tongue."

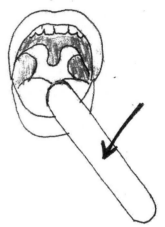

tongue blade
\'tʌŋ bleɪd\ a flat piece of wood
used to hold the tongue down during
examination of the throat SYN: tongue
depressor.
"A **tongue blade** looks like a popsicle
stick."

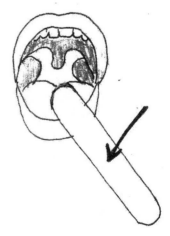

tongue depressor
\tʌŋ də-'pre-sɜ:\ a flat piece of wood
used to hold the tongue down during
examination of the throat SYN: tongue
blade.
"A **tongue depressor** is used when the
doctor says, 'Say ahhh.'"

tonsils
\'tɒn-səlz\ two masses of lymphoid
tissue that lie on each side of the throat
"The surgery to remove **tonsils** is called
a *tonsillectomy*."

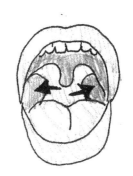

too numerous to count (*abbrev.*)
\tɪ:-en-tɪ:-'sɪ:\ a microbiology lab
description
"The cells on the slide were **TNTC**
under the microscope."

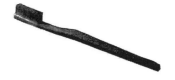

toothbrush
\'tu:ɵ-brʌʃ\ a utensil with bristles for
cleaning the teeth and mouth
"The hospital can provide a **toothbrush**
for you."

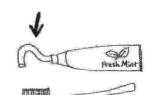

toothpaste
\'tu:ɵ-peɪst\ a paste for cleaning the
teeth
"Most **toothpaste** is mint flavored."

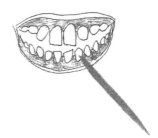

toothpick
\'tu:ɵ-pɪk\ a pointed instrument that
removes food stuck between the teeth
"Do you have a **toothpick** or some
dental floss?"

torso

\'tɔ:-səʊ\ the main part of the body exluding the arms and legs SYN: trunk. "Some viral infections can cause a rash on the **torso**."

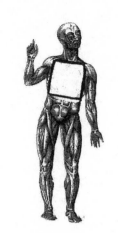

total iron-binding capacity (*abbrev.*)

\tɪ:-ɑɪ-bɪ:-'sɪ:\ a blood test "**TIBC** is a blood test done to help diagnose iron-deficiency anemia."

TIBC

total parenteral nutrition (*abbrev.*)

\tɪ:-pɪ:-'en\ nutrition given intravenously "The patient with a bowel obstruction was started on **TPN**."

TPN

tourniquet

\'tɜ:-nə-kɪt\ a device used to bind a limb and cut off blood flow "When fingers become swollen, a ring will act like a **tourniquet** if not removed."

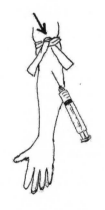

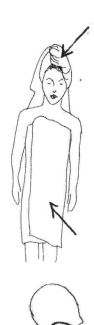

towel
\'tɑʊ-əl\ an absorbent cloth or paper for wiping or drying
"Wrap a **towel** around the patient's wet hair to avoid chilling."

trachea
\'treɪ-kɪ:-ə\ the firm tube stretching from the pharynx to the main bronchials SYN: windpipe.
"A tension pneumothorax can cause deviation of the **trachea**."
tracheal (*adj.*)

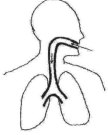

transient ischemic attack (*abbrev.*)
\tɪ:-ɑɪ-'eɪ\ a temporary lack of blood flow to the brain
"A carotid ultrasound was done on the patient with a hx of **TIA**."

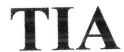

transurethral resection of the prostate
(*abbrev.*)
\tɜ:p\ a urological surgical procedure
"The patient had a **TURP** done due to urinary retention."

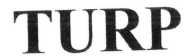

trapezius
\træ-ʹpɪ:-zɪ:-əs\ a flat, triangular
muscle covering the back of the neck
and shoulder
"Heavy lifting can strain the **trapezius**
muscle."

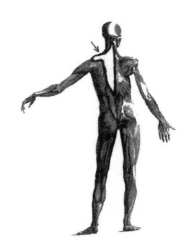

trapezoid
\ʹtræ-pə-zɔɪd\ a four-sided figure with
only two sides parallel
"Some pills are shaped like a
trapezoid."

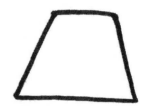

trash can
\ʹtræʃ-kæn\ a receptacle for waste
materials
"Some **trash cans** are designated for
recyclable items only."
cans (*pl.*)

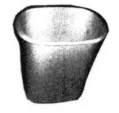

triangle
\ʹtrɑɪ-æŋ-əl\ a polygon having three
sides
"A **triangle** with an exlcamation point
inside is used as a caution sign."
triangular (*adj.*)

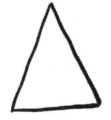

the symbol for **treatment**
\ʹtrɪ:t-mənt\ or **therapy**
\ʹθeə-ə-pɪ:\ a medical intervention
"Pt. receiving whirlpool **tx** BID."

Tx

triceps
\'trɑɪ-seps\ the muscle on the back of
the upper arm
"Push-ups can strengthen the **triceps**
muscles."

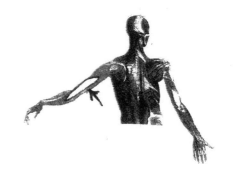

tricuspid valve
\trɑɪ-'kʌs-pɪd vælv\ the heart valve
between the right atrium and right
ventricle
SYN: right atrioventricular valve.
"A **tricuspid valve** is named for its
three leaflets."

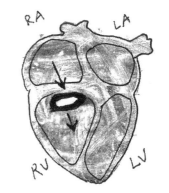

tripod
\'trɑɪ-pɒd\ having three legs; a position
assumed that resembles a tripod
"The COPD patient was sitting in a
tripod position."

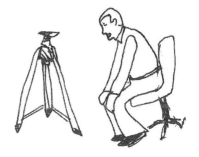

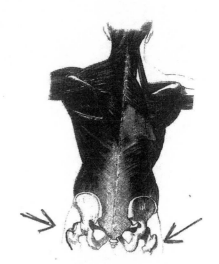

trochanter
\trəʊ-'kæn-tɜ:\ the part of the femur
that protrudes out at the hip
"Bedridden patients are susceptible
to pressue ulcers forming in the
trochanter region."

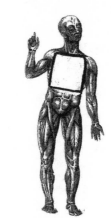

trunk
\trʌnk\ the main part of the body
excluding the arms and legs SYN: torso.
"*Truncal obesity* refers to fat deposits
around the **trunk** area."
truncal (*adj.*)

tuberculosis (*abbrev.*)
\tɪ:-'bɪ:\ an infectious disease that
affects the lungs and other organs
"Healthcare workers are required to
have regular **TB** tests."

TB

Tuesday (*abbrev.*)
\'tu:z-deɪ\ the third day of the week
"The presidential election is held on a
Tues."

Tues.

tweezers
\'twɪ:-z3:z\ a metal instrument used for grasping or manipulating small items "I need some **tweezers** to remove that last suture."

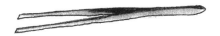

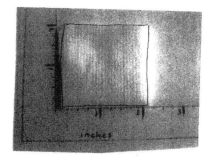

2 × 2
\'tu:-bɑɪ-tu:\ a piece of sterile gauze approximately two inches square "Put a **2 × 2** over that IV site please."

Chapter Twenty One

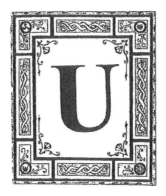

Uu \ju:\
The letter *U* is the twenty-first letter of the English alphabet.

U is for *unicorn*. \'ju:-nɪ-kɔ:n\
"The **unicorn** is a mythological creature."

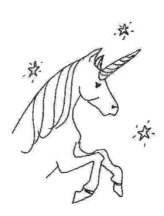

ulna
\'ʌl-nə\ the longer bone of the forearm
that forms the elbow
"The forearm bones are the **ulna** and
radius."

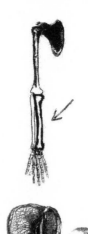

umbilical cord
\ʌm-'bɪ-lə-kəl kɔ:d\ the attachment
connecting the fetus to the placenta
"The father was in the delivery room
and cut the **umbilical cord**."

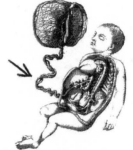

umbilicus
\ʌm-'bɪ-lə-kəs\ the abdominal scar
from the umbilical cord
SYN: belly button, navel.
"An **umbilical** hernia can cause the
abdomen to bulge out."
umbilical (*adj.*)

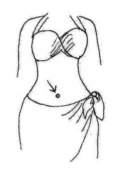

umbrella
\ʌm-'bre-lə\ a collapsible shade to
protect against the elements
"There are plastic bags at the entrance
for your wet **umbrella**."

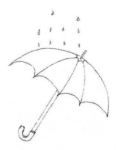

underarm
\'ʌn-dɜ:-ɑ:m\ the area beneath the shoulder between the arm and thorax
SYN: axilla, armpit.
"Do you have any **underarm** deodorant that I can use after I bathe?"

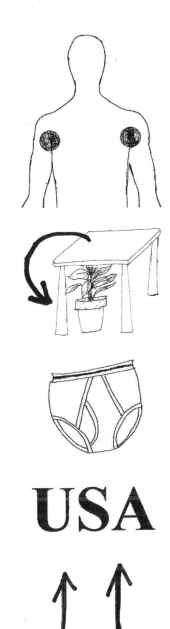

underneath
\ʌn-dɜ:-'nɪ:θ\ under or below an object or surface
"The plant is **underneath** the table."

underwear
\'ʌn-dɜ:-weə\ clothing worn next to the skin under other clothing
"The patient prefers to keep his **underwear** on."

unstable angina (*abbrev.*)
\'ʌn-steɪ-bəl 'æn-dʒə-nə\ a type of chest pain
"**USA** may be treated with nitrates"

up
\ʌp\ in a higher point or direction
"The opposite of **up** is down."

upper respiratory infection (*abbrev.*)
\ju:-ɑ:-'ɑɪ\ acute infections of the nose,
sinuses, and throat
"A cold is one type of **URI**."

URI

urinal
\'jɜ:-ə-nəl\ a urine receptacle
"Another name for **urinal** is *pee bottle*
or *jug*."

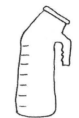

urinary tract infection (*abbrev.*)
\ju:-tɪ:-'ɑɪ\ an infection in the kidneys,
ureters, or bladder
"An untreated **UTI** can progress to
urosepsis and shock."

UTI

urine output (*abbrev.*)
\'jɜ:-ɪn 'aʊt-pʊt\ a measure of urine
production and excretion
"A **UO** of < 30 ml/hr. should be
reported to the doctor."

U.O.

uterus
\'ju:-də-rɪs\ the womb of a female
mammal
"A hysterectomy procedure removes the
uterus."

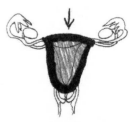

uvula
\'ju:-vju:-lə\ the piece of flesh that
hangs in the back of the throat above the
base of the tongue
"One symptom of epiglottitis is a
swollen **uvula**."

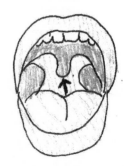

Chapter Twenty Two

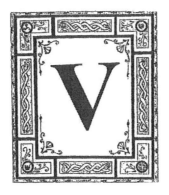

Vv \vɪ:\
The letter *V* is the twenty-second letter of the English alphabet.

V is for *violin.* \vɑɪ-ə-'lɪn\
"Another name for **violin** is *fiddle.*"

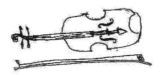

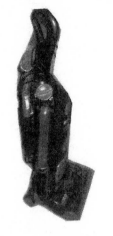

vacuum cleaner
\'væk-ju:m 'klɪ:-nɜ:\ a household
appliance for cleaning floors or carpet
by suction
"**Vacuum cleaners** create a lot of noise
in the hospital."
cleaners (*pl.*)

vancomycin-resistant enterococcus
(*abbrev.*)
\vɪ:-ɑ:-'ɪ:\ a type of antibiotic-resistant
microorganism
"He is in isolation for **VRE** in the
urine."

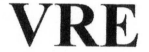

vase
\veɪs\ *or* \vɒz\ an ornamental container
used to hold flowers
"Do you have a **vase** to put these
flowers in?"

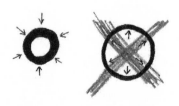

vasoconstriction
\veɪ-zəʊ-kʌn-'strɪk-ʃən\ a decrease in
the diameter of blood vessels
"A vasopressor induces
vasoconstriction to raise blood
pressure."

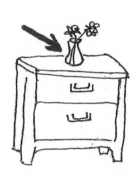

vasodilation
\veɪ-zəʊ-dɑɪ-'leɪ-ʃən\ an increase in the diameter of blood vessels
"Nitrates induce **vasodilation** to lower blood pressure."

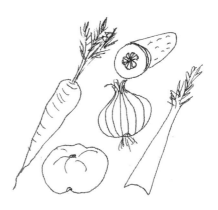

vegetables
\'vedʒ-tə-bəlz\ edible plants grown for food
"I need to eat more **vegetables** for roughage."

Venereal Disease Research Laboratories (*abbrev.*)
\vɪ:-dɪ:-ɑ:-'el\ a blood test for syphilis
"An RPR test is similar to a **VDRL** test."

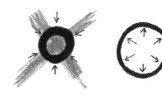

venous thromboembolism (*abbrev.*)
\vɪ:-tɪ:-'ɪ:\ a clot that blocks a blood vessel SYN: blood clot.
"**VTE** prophylaxis may include blood thinners."

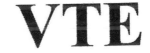

ventilator
\'ven-tɪ-leɪ-dɜ:\ a machine used to assist ventilation and oxygenation
SYN: life support, respirator.
"The patient with acute respiratory failure was placed on a **ventilator**."

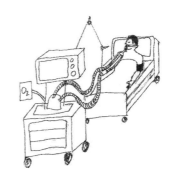

ventricle
\'ven-trɪ-kəl\ one of two lower
chambers of the heart
"She has right **ventricular**
hypertrophy."
ventricular (*adj.*)

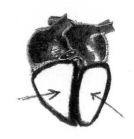

ventricular fibrillation
\ven-'trɪk-ju:-lɜ: fɪ-brɪ-'leɪ-ʃən\ a
condition of quivering of the bottom
chambers of the heart
"The patient collapsed and was found
to be in **ventricular fibrillation** on the
monitor."

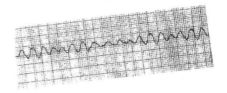

ventricular fibrillation (*abbrev.*)
\vɪ:-'ef\ a cardiac arrhythmia
"The patient in **VF** needs immediate
defibrillation."

VF

ventricular tachycardia
\ven-'trɪk-ju:-lɜ: tæ-kɪ-'kɑ:-dɪ:-ə\ a
rapid rhythm originating in the lower
chambers of the heart that can be fatal
"The patient with low potassium and
magnesium had runs of **ventricular
tachycardia**."

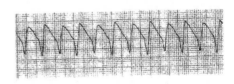

ventricular tachycardia (*abbrev.*)
\vɪ:-'tɪ:\ a cardiac arrhythmia
"The patient has been having frequent
runs of **VT**."

VT

vest restaint
\vest rɪ-'streɪnt\ a garment worn on the torso with ties to secure the patient to a bed frame or chair
"A commonly used brand name for a **vest restraint** is *Posey® vest* \pəʊ-zɪ: vest\."

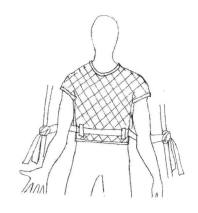

vial
\vɑɪl\ a small glass bottle for medicines or liquids
"Insulin can be stored in a multidose **vial**."

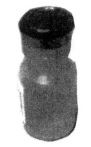

vital signs (*abbrev.*)
\'vɑɪ-dəl sɑɪnz\ signs of life that include pulse, respirations, and blood pressure
"The patient's **vital signs** have been stable."

voice box
\'vɔɪs bɒks\ the vocal cords inside the larynx SYN: larynx, Adam's apple.
"You can't talk because the tube is in your **voice box**."

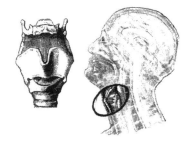

Chapter Twenty Three

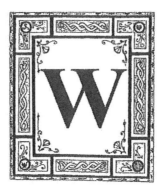

Ww \\'dʌ-bəl-ju:\\
The letter *W* is the twenty-third letter of the English alphabet.

W is for *water*. \\'wɒ-dɜ:\\
"You can lead a horse to **water**, but you can't make it drink."

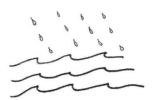

waist

\weɪst\ the narrowed part of the body
between the thorax and the hips
"Abdominal girth is measured at the
waist."

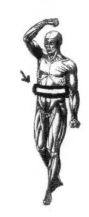

walk

\wɒk\ to move along on foot SYN:
ambulate.
"The surgeon would like you to **walk** at
least 3 times a day."

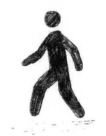

walker

\'wɒ-kɜ:\ a framework designed to
support a person while walking
"The patient ambulates with a **walker**."

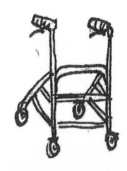

wallet

\'wɒ-lət\ a folded pocketbook designed
to hold cards and money
"I keep my driver's license in my
wallet."

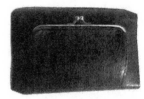

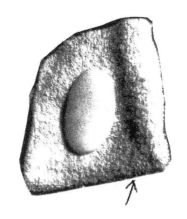

washcloth
\'wɒʃ-klɒɵ\ a small towel used to wash
the face and body
"Here's a warm **washcloth** for your face
and hands."

watch
\wɒtʃ\ a portable clock that is worn or
carried
"He wears his **watch** on his left wrist."

the formula for **water**
\eɪtʃ-tu:-'əʊ\ the principal constituent of
all body fluids
"Free **H₂O** flushes Q6h."

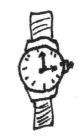

$$H2O$$

water pitcher
\'wɒ-dɜ: 'pɪ-tʃɜ:\ a container to hold
drinking water
"Would you please refill my **water
pitcher**?"

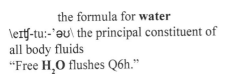

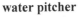

Wednesday (*abbrev.*)
\'wenz-deɪ\ the fourth day of the week
"**Wed.** is called *hump day* because it's
in the middle of the week."

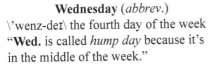

$$\textbf{Wed.}$$

weed
\wɪːd\ marijuana SYN: pot.
"The patient said he smokes **weed** every day."

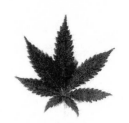

week
\wɪːk\ a seven-day cycle beginning with Sunday and ending with Saturday
"There are seven days in a **week**."

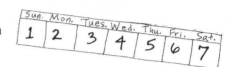

wet floor
\wet 'flɔː\ a caution sign to prevent falls
"Put up **wet floor** signs when you are mopping."

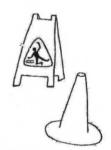

wheat cereal
\wɪːt 'sɪə-ɪ:-əl\ a hot food made of wheat farina and served at breakfast
"A common brand name for **wheat cereal** served in the hospital is *Cream of Wheat* ® \krɪːm ʌv 'wɪːt\."

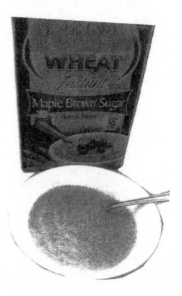

wheelchair
\'wɪː-l-ʧeə\ a chair mounted on wheels
that is used to transport people
"Patient transported to car via
wheelchair."

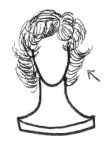

wig
\wɪg\ a covering for the head made of
real or synthetic hair
"The patient prefers to keep her **wig**
on."

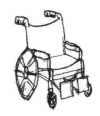

window
\'wɪn-dəʊ\ an opening in a wall of a
building to let in light and air
"Please open the **window** for some
fresh air."

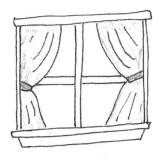

windpipe
\'wɪn-pɑɪp\ the trachea SYN: airway.
"Aspiration means your drink went
down your **windpipe**."

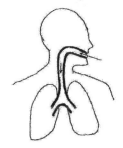

within defined limits (*abbrev.*)
\wɪθ-'ɪn də-'fɑɪnd 'lɪ-mətz\ normal
SYN: WNL.
"Assessment **WDL**."

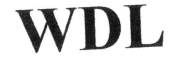

within normal limits (*abbrev.*)
\wɪɵ-'ɪn 'nɔ:-məl 'lɪ-mətz\ normal
SYN: WDL.
"Abdominal assessment **WNL**."

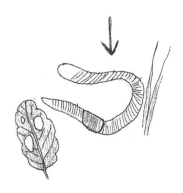

worm
\wɜ:m\ earthworm; any small elongated
soft-bodied animal; insect larva
"Test the stool for intestinal **worms**."
worms (*pl.*)

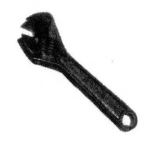

wrench
\rentʃ\ a tool for holding or turning an
object
"When things don't go as planned a
person may say, 'well, this really throws
a **wrench** in the works'."

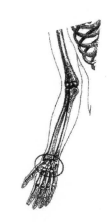

wrist
\rɪst\ the joint between the hand and the
forearm SYN: carpus.
"Carpal-tunnel surgery involves the
wrist."

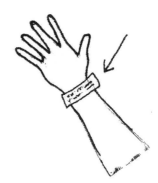

wristband
\'rɪs-bænd\ nameband with patient
identification SYN: nameband.
"I'm going to scan your **wristband**."

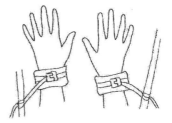

wrist restraints
\'rɪst rə-'streɪntz\ soft ties placed on the
wrists for safety
"**Wrist restraints** applied to prevent
extubation."

Chapter Twenty Four

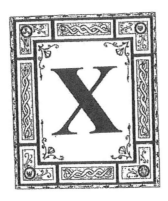

Xx \eks\
The letter *X* is the twenty-fourth letter of the English alphabet.

X is for *xylophone*. \'zɑɪ-lə-fəʊn\
"The **xylophone** is a percussion instrument."

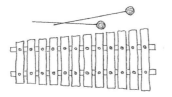

xiphoid process
\'zɑɪ-fɔɪd 'prɒ-səs\ the proximal end of the sternum
"Avoid pressure on the **xiphoid process** during chest compressions."

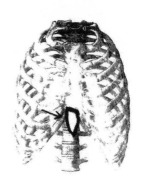

x-ray
\'eks-reɪ\ a radiologic picture
"*X-ray* is another name for the radiology department."

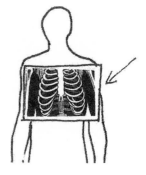

Chapter Twenty Five

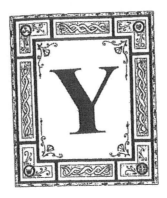

Yy \waɪ\
The letter *Y* is the twenty-fifth letter of the English alphabet.

Y is for *yardstick.* \'jɑ:d-stɪk\ a graduated measuring stick, three feet long
"A **yardstick** is almost the same length as one meter."

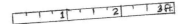

Yankauer
\'jæn-kɑʊ-ɜ:\ a hard plastic oral suction catheter
"A **Yankauer** is used to clear oral secretions."

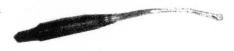
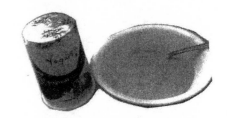

yogurt
\'jəʊ-gɜ:t\ a cultured milk product
"Eating **yogurt** may help maintain balanced intestinal flora."

Chapter Twenty Six

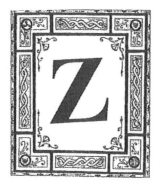

Zz \zɪ:\
The letter *Z* is the twenty-sixth and final letter of the English alphabet.

Z is for *zero*. \'zɪ:-rəʊ\ the absence of all magnitude or quantity
"Another word for **zero** is *nil*."

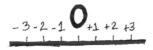

zigzag
\'zɪg zæg\ having short, sharp turns or angles
"He was **zigzagging** down the hall."

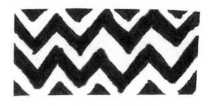

the symbol for the element **zinc**
\zɪːnk\ refer to the periodic table of the elements
"Some people believe taking **zinc** can help prevent colds."

References

Merriam-Webster. 1996. *Merriam-Webster's Collegiate Dictionary*, 10th ed. Springfield, Massachusetts: Merriam-Webster.

Venes, Donald, ed. 2005. *Taber's Cyclopedic Medical Dictionary*, 20th ed. Philadelphia: F.A. Davis Company.

Index

A

ABD, 18
abdomen, 18, 43
abdominal, 18
abdominal aortic aneurysm, 18
abduction, 18, 22
ABG, 32
above, 19
above-the-knee amputation, 19
ac, 28
ACEI, 27
acetabular, 19
acetabulum, 19
acetylsalicylic acid, 20
Ace Wrap®, 99
Achilles tendon, 20
acid-fast bacilli, 20
ACL, 28
ACLS, 23
acquired immunodeficiency syndrome, 20
acromion process, 20, 218
ACS, 21
activities of daily living, 21
acute coronary syndrome, 21
acute lymphocytic leukemia, 21
acute myeloid leukemia, 21
acute myocardial infarction, 21
acute renal failure, 21
acute tubular necrosis, 21
ADA, 25
Adam's apple, 22, 149, 259
adduction, 18, 22
ADH, 29
ADHD, 33

adhesive bandage, 22
adipose tissue, 22
ADLs, 21
adrenal glands, 23
adult respiratory distress syndrome, 23
advanced cardiac life support, 23
AED, 35
aerosol mask, 23
AF, 33-34
AFB, 20
AG, 27
AICD, 35
AIDS, 20
airway, 24, 265
AKA, 19
alanine aminotransferase, 24
albuterol, 168
ALL, 21
alpha, 24
ALS, 26
ALT, 24
alveolar, 24
alveoli, 24
alveolus, 24
AMA, 23
Ambu bag, 24, 39
ambulance, 25
ambulate, 25, 262
ambulatory, 25
American Diabetes Association, 25
American Medical Association, 23
AMI, 21
AML, 21
ammonia, 25
amniotic fluid, 25

ampule, 26
amputation, 26
amyotrophic lateral sclerosis, 26
ANA, 29
aneurysm, 26
angioplasty, 27
angiotensin-converting enzyme inhibitor, 27
angry, 27
anion gap, 27
ankle, 27, 233
ante cibum, 28
antecubital fossa, 28
ante meridiem, 28
anterior, 28
anterior cruciate ligament, 28
anterior-posterior, 29
antibiotic-resistant microorganisms, 29
antibodies, 29
antidiuretic hormone, 29
antinuclear antibody, 29
anus, 29
aorta, 30
aortic stenosis, 30
aortic valve, 30
AP, 29
appendicitis, 30
appendix, 30
apple, 17
applesauce, 30
arch, 31
ARDS, 23
ARF, 21
arm, 31
ARM, 29
armpit, 31
arrow, 32
arterial blood gas, 32
artery, 32
arthritis, 88
ASA, 20
ASAP, 33
ascites, 32
aspartate aminotransferase, 32
aspirate, 33

aspirin, 20, 172
as soon as possible, 33
AST, 32
atelectasis, 33
atherosclerosis, 34
ATN, 21
atria, 33-34
atrial, 33-34, 195
atrial fibrillation, 33-34
atrioventricular block, 34
atrium, 34
Aug., 34
August, 34
auricle, 35
auscultation, 35
automated external defibrillator, 35
automated implanted cardiac defibrillator, 35
AVB, 34
axilla, 36, 253
axillae, 36
axillary, 36

B

baby, 37, 110
baby bottle, 38
baby food, 38
bacillus, 20
back, 38
backbone, 38, 224
backpack, 39
BAER, 52
balance, 66, 134
bald, 39
balloon, 39
ballpoint pen, 39
banana, 40
bandage, 40, 95
bandage scissors, 40
Bandaid®, 14, 22
barium, 40
basic life support, 40
basic metabolic panel, 40
basilic vein, 41

basin, 41
bassinet, 41
batteries, 41
beard, 41
bed, 42
bedpan, 42
bedridden, 248
bedside commode, 42
bedspread, 42
bee, 42
beef, 43
belladonna and opium, 38
belly, 43, 226
belly button, 43, 168, 252
below, 43
below-the-knee amputation, 44
belt, 44
beta, 44
Betadine®, 194
beveled, 45
bicarbonate, 45
biceps, 45
bicuspid valve, 45, 162
bicycle, 46
bifurcation, 46
bigeminy, 46
big toe, 46, 56, 124
bike, 46
biohazard, 46
biopsy, 46
bladder, 47
blanket, 47
bleach, 47
blink, 47
blood clot, 48
blood pressure, 51
blood pressure cuff, 48
blood sugar, 48, 86
blood urea nitrogen, 48
BM, 48
BMI, 49
BMP, 40
B&O, 38
bobby pins, 48
body mass index, 49

boiling, 49
boots, 49
bottle, 49
bottom, 50, 57
bow, 50
bowel, 50
bowel movement, 48
bowel sounds, 48, 50
bowl, 50
box, 51
boxer shorts, 54
BP, 51
BP cuff, 48
bra, 51
bracelet, 51
brachial, 51
braids, 52
brain, 52, 66
brainstem, 52, 87
brainstem auditory evoked response, 52
bread, 52, 80
break, 53
breastbone, 53, 226
breastfeeding, 53
briefs, 54
broken, 53
bronchials, 54
bronchodilator, 168
broom, 54
bruise, 54, 132
brush, 54, 124
BS, 48
BSC, 42, 75, 194
bucket, 55
Buck's traction, 55
bulb drain, 55
bulb syringe, 55
BUN, 48
bundle branch block, 56
bunion, 56
burn, 56
butter, 56
buttocks, 50, 57

C

C, 62
CA, 62
Ca++, 61
CABG, 79
CaCl, 60
caduceus, 60
caffeine, alcohol, pepper, aspirin-free, 60
cake, 60
calcaneus, 20, 60, 127
calcium, 61
calcium chloride, 60
calendar, 61
calf, 61
call bell, 61
call light, 61
calves, 61
camera, 61
cancer, 62
cane, 62
cannabinoids, 193
cap, 109, 134
CAPA-free, 60
capillary refill, 72
capsule, 62
carbohydrates, 62
carbon dioxide, 63
cardiac output, 63
cardiopulmonary resuscitation, 63
carotid, 63
carpus, 63, 266
cast, 64
cat, 59
cataract, 64
catheter, 64
cath tip syringe, 64
CBC, 76
cc, 82
cecum, 65
celiac disease, 52
centimeter, 65
central nervous system, 65
central venous pressure, 65
cerebellum, 66

cerebral, 26, 52, 66, 76, 86, 116
cerebral aneurysm, 26, 65
cerebral palsy, 66
cerebral perfusion pressure, 66
cerebrospinal fluid, 66, 154, 223
cerebrum, 52, 66
cervical collar, 67
cervical spine, 67, 169
cervix, 67
chair, 67
change, 68, 74
   coins, 68
   delta, 88
chest, 238
chest of drawers, 68, 95
chest tube, 68-69
chest-tube clamp, 69
chest x-ray, 69
chewing gum, 69, 121
CHF, 77
chin, 70
chloride, 70
CHO, 62
Christmas Day, 86
chronic kidney disease, 70
chronic lymphocytic leukemia, 70
chronic myelogenous leukemia, 70
chronic obstructive pulmonary disease, 71
cigarettes, 71, 151
circle, 71
circle of Willis, 71
circulation, 72
circumflex artery, 72
cirrhosis, 32, 103
CIS, 76
CKD, 70
Cl-, 70
clavicle, 72, 75
clipboard, 72
CLL, 70
clock, 73
CML, 70
CMV, 83
CMX, 72
CNS, 65

CO, 62
CO2, 63
coat, 73
coccyx, 232
cochlea, 74
cochlear, 74
coffee, 74
coins, 68, 74
collar bone, 72
collarbone, 75
colostomy, 75
commode, 42, 75, 194
complete blood count, 76
computed tomography, 76
computer information systems, 76
computerized provider order entry, 76
computer on wheels, 76
cone, 76
confidentiality, 127
congestive heart failure, 77
conjunctiva, 77
conjunctival, 77
consistent carbohydrate diet, 25
continuous positive air pressure, 77
contracture, 77
cookies, 78
COPD, 71
cornea, 47, 78
corneal stimulation, 47
coronary artery bypass graft, 78-79
cotton-tipped applicator, 79
cow, 43, 79
COW, 76
CP, 66
CPAP, 77
CPAP mask, 79
CPK, 80
CPOE, 76
CPP, 66
CPR, 63
crab, 79
crackers, 80
cramping, 61, 136
cranial, 80
cranium, 80

crash cart, 80
C-reactive protein, 80
Cream of Wheat®, 264
creatine phosphokinase, 80
crib, 80
cross, 81, 295
crotch, 81, 121
CRP, 80
crutch, 81
crutches, 81
C&S, 82
CSF, 66
CT, 76
cube, 81
cubic centimeter, 82
culture, 82
culture and sensitivity, 82
cup, 82
curved, 82
cut, 83
cuticle, 83
CVP, 65
CXR, 69
cyanosis, 152
cylinder, 83
cylindrical, 83
cytomegalovirus, 83

D

D5W, 90
D10W, 90
D50, 89
date of birth, 86
daytime, 86
DBP, 91
D&C, 92
Dec., 86
December, 86
decerebrate, 86
deciliter, 86
decimal point, 87
decorticate, 87
decrease, 87
deep vein thrombosis, 87

defibrillator, 87
degenerative joint disease, 88
dehydration, 21
delirium tremens, 88
delta, 88
deltoid, 88
dentition, 88, 234
denture cleaner, 89
denture cup, 89
dentures, 89
depolarization, 195, 200
dermatomes, 89
diabetes mellitus, 90
diabetic ketoacidosis, 90
diagnosis-related group, 90
diagonal, 90
diameter, 90
diaper, 91
diaphragm, 91
diastolic blood pressure, 91
DIC, 93
dicrotic notch, 91
digestive tract, 91
digits, 92
dilation, 92
dilation and curettage, 92
diphtheria, pertussis, tetanus, 92
disinfectant, 47
disk, 92
dislocation, 93
disseminated intravascular coagulation, 93
distal, 93
diverticula, 93
diverticulitis, 93
diverticulum, 93
DJD, 88
DKA, 90
dl, 86
DM, 90
DNR, 94
dollar sign, 94
do not resuscitate, 94
doughnut, 94
down, 94
DPAHC, 96

DPT, 92
drain, 94
dressing, 95
DRG, 90
drink, 95
drip, 95
drop, 95
DTs, 88
duodenal, 95
duodenum, 95
dustpan, 96

E

ear, 98
    nose, and throat, 98
ear lobe, 197
earlobe, 98
earplugs, 98
earrings, 98
EBL, 103
EBV, 102
ECG, 100
echocardiogram, 99
ED, 101
EEG, 100
Efferdent®, 89
eggs, 97
eighth, 99
EKG, 99-100
elastic bandage, 99
elbow, 99
electrical, 100
electricity, 100
electrocardiogram, 100
electrodes, 99-100
electroencephalogram, 100
electrophysiology, 100
elevate, 101
elevator, 101, 112
eleventh, 15, 143, 172
EM, 102
emergency department, 101
emergency medical technician, 101
emergency room, 101

emesis basin, 101, 224
emphysema, 238
endotracheal tube, 101
end-stage renal disease, 102
end-tidal carbon dioxide, 102
ENT, 98
enteral, 168
entrance, 102
EP, 100
epi, 102
epiglottitis, 254
epinephrine, 102
epistaxis, 172
EPO, 103
Epstein-Barr virus, 102
equal sign, 102
ER, 101
erythrocyte sedimentation rate, 102
erythromycin, 102
ESBL, 104
esophageal, 103
esophageal varices, 103
esophagus, 103
ESR, 102
estimated blood loss, 103
estimated time of arrival, 103
E&T, 103
ETA, 103
ETCO2, 102
ethyl alcohol, 103
ETOH, 103
ET tube, 101
evaluate and treat, 103
evening, 193
every other day, 200
exclamation point, 104
exit, 104
extend, 104
extended-spectrum beta-lactamase, 104
extension, 104
eyebrows, 105
eyelashes, 105
eyelids, 105

F

FA, 114
facial droop, 108
fallopian tubes, 108
fan, 108
farina, 108
Father's Day, 141
faucets, 220
Fe, 136
feather, 109
Feb., 109
February, 109
fecal occult blood test, 109
feeding pump, 109
feet, 114
felt-tip pen, 109
femoral, 110
femur, 110
FeSO4, 228
fetus, 110
fever, 110
fever of unknown origin, 111
FFP, 115
fibrinogen, 93
fibula, 111
fiddle, 255
fifth, 111
FiO2, 115
fire, 56, 112, 115, 122
fire alarm, 112
fire extinguisher, 112
first, 112
fish, 107
fist, 113
flashlight, 113
flex, 44, 113
flowers, 113
flow meter, 113
FOB, 102, 114
FOBT, 109
Foley® catheter, 64
follow-up, 114
fontanel, 80
foot, 114

foot of bed, 114
forearm, 114
forehead, 114
fork, 115
forty-five degree angle, 176
fossae, 28
4 × 4, 115
fourth, 115
fractional concentration of inspired oxygen, 115
fracture, 53
freezing, 49
fresh frozen plasma, 115
Fri., 116
Friday, 116
frontal lobe, 116
frown, 116
fruit, 116
F/U, 114
funny bone, 116
FUO, 111
furniture, 42, 68, 95

G

gallbladder, 118
gamma, 118
gangrene, 26
gastric banding, 226
gastroesophageal reflux disease, 118
gauze, 119
GCS, 119
GERD, 118
GFR, 119
GI bleeding, 20
Glasgow Coma Scale, 119
glass, 119
glomerular filtration rate, 119
gluteal, 120
gluten, 52
goiter, 239
golf ball, 120
gonads, 120, 236
grimace, 121
groin, 81, 121

gtt, 95
guaiac, 109
guitar, 117
gum, 69, 121
gums, 122
gut, 50

H

H2O, 263
H2O2, 130
hairbrush, 54, 124
Halloween, 177
hallux, 46, 124
halo, 124
hammer, 124
hamstrings, 125
hand, 125
handheld nebulizer, 125
happy face, 126, 222
hat, 126
HCO3, 45
head, 126
head of bed, 126
headphones, 127
Health Insurance Portability and Accountability Act, 127
hearing aids, 126-27
heart, 127
heel, 127
height, 128
hematoma, 124
hemispheres, 52, 66
hemoglobin and hematocrit, 128
hemostat, 128
hemotoxins, 222
hexagon, 128
hexagonal, 128
HHN, 125
hiccups, 91
high Fowler's position, 208
HIPAA, 127
hips, 128
history, 129
history and physical, 129

HOB, 126
HOH, 126
hora somni, 129
hospital gown, 129
hot, 129
H&P, 129
HS, 129
ht., 128
HTN, 130
humerus, 130
hump day, 263
hx, 129
hydrogen peroxide, 130
hypertension, 130
hyponatremia, 222
hypophosphatemia, 188
hysterectomy, 254

I

IABP, 135
IBS, 136
ice cream, 131
ICP, 135
ICU, 135
I&D, 133
IDDM, 134
idiopathic thrombocytopenia purpura, 132
IJ, 135
ileal, 132
ileum, 132
incentive spirometer, 132
incision and drainage, 133
increase, 133
Independence Day, 141
index finger, 133
infant, 53, 55, 170
inhaler, 134, 159
insomnia, 129
instep, 134
insulin-dependent diabetes mellitus, 134
insulin syringe, 134
intake and output, 134
intensive care unit, 135
internal jugular, 135

intestines, 50, 135
intra-aortic balloon pump, 135
intracranial pressure, 135
intravenous, 135
intravenous fluids, 136
I&O, 134
iodine, 136
ion, 61, 70, 156, 222
iron, 136
irritable bowel syndrome, 136
IS, 132
ischial tuberosity, 136
isolation, 21, 29, 104, 137, 157, 256
isolation gown, 137
ITP, 132, 224
IV, 135
IVF, 136
IV pole, 137

J

jacket, 140
Jackson-Pratt bulb drain, 140
Jan., 140
January, 140
JCAHO, 140
jejunostomy tube, 140
jejunum, 140
jewelry, 139
Joint Commission on the Accreditation of
        Healthcare Organizations, 140
JP drain, 140
J-tube, 140
jug, 254
jugular vein, 141
jugular venous distention, 141
July, 141
June, 141
JVD, 141

K

K+, 193
kangaroo, 143
KCl, 193

Kelly clamp, 144
ketchup, 144
kidneys, 144
ureters, and bladder, 144
knee, 145
kneecap, 145, 185
knife, 145
knives, 145
KOH, 194
KPO4, 161, 194
KUB, 144
kyphosis, 146

L

labor, 67, 148
labor and delivery, 148
Labor Day, 215
laceration, 83, 148
lactate dehydrogenase, 148
lactated Ringer's, 148
LAD, 150
ladder, 148
lamp, 149
laryngitis, 149
larynx, 22, 149, 259
laser, 78
lat, 150, 176
lateral, 149
lb., 194
L&D, 148, 176
LDH, 148
left anterior descending artery, 150
left main artery, 150
legs, 150, 153
LEs, 153
less than, 150
level, 150
level of consciousness, 151
LFTs, 152
lido, 151
life support, 151
lightbulb, 147, 149
lighter, 151, 212
lip balm, 151

lips, 152
lipstick, 152
LIS, 153
liver, 152
liver function tests, 152
lobectomy, 68
lobster, 153
LOC, 151
Lopez valve, 153
Lou Gehrig's disease, 26
lower extremities, 153
low intermittent suction, 153
LP, 154
LR, 148
Luer lock, 153
lumbar puncture, 154
lumen, 90
lungs, 154

M

magnet, 156
magnetic field, 156
magnetic resonance angiography, 156
magnetic resonance imaging, 156
magnifying glass, 156
makeup, 156
malleolus, 159, 233
Mar., 157
MAR, 158
March, 157
mask, 157
mastectomy, 48
matches, 157
May, 157
mcg, 160
MD, 158
MDI, 159
measles, mumps, rubella, 157
measuring tape, 158
med, 158-59
med cup, 158
medial, 159
medical doctor, 158
MedicAlert® bracelet, 159

medical record number, 159
medication, 159
Medication Administration Record, 158
Memorial Day, 157
meningitis, 66
mEq, 161
metered-dose inhaler, 159
methicillin-resistant *Staphylococcus aureus*, 160
metoprolol, 44
mg, 160-61
Mg++, 156
MI, 163
micrograms, 160
microscope, 160
middle finger, 160
midnight, 161
milk, 161
milliequivalents, 161
milligrams, 161
millimeters of mercury, 161
millimoles, 161
mitral valve, 45, 162
mmHg, 161
MMR, 157
MN, 161
mo., 162
Mon., 162
Monday, 162
money, 68, 162
mononucleosis, 102
month, 162
moon, 155
mop, 162
morning, 28
morphine sulfate, 163
motor vehicle accident, 163
mouse, 163
MRA, 156
MRI, 156
MRN, 159
MRSA, 160
MS, 163
multiple sclerosis, 163
MVA, 163
myocardial infarction, 21, 163

N

Na+, 222
NaCl, 212, 222
nail clippers, 166
nail polish, 166
nameband, 166, 267
napkin, 166
narcs, 166
nares, 167
naris, 167
nasal cannula, 167
nasogastric tube, 168
navel, 43, 168
NC, 167
neb, 168
nebulizer, 125, 168
neck, 67, 169
necklace, 169
needle, 169
neonatal intensive care unit, 169
neuro, 52
neurotoxins, 222
NGT, 168
NH3, 25
NIBP, 171
NICU, 169
NIDDM, 171
night, 170
nighttime, 170
ninety-degree angle, 208
ninety degrees, 27
ninth, 170
nipple, 170
nitrates, 253, 257
nitroglycerin, 170
NKA, 171
noc, 170
nocturnal, 170
no known allergies, 171
noninsulin-dependent diabetes mellitus, 171
non per os, 171
nonrebreather, 171
nonrebreather mask, 171
non-STEMI, 172

nonsteroidal anti-inflammatory drug, 172
normal saline, 222
north, 165
nose, 172
nothing by mouth, 171
Nov., 172
November, 172
NPH, 173
NPH insulin, 173
NPO, 171
NSAIDS, 172
NTG, 170
nuts, 173

O

oatmeal, 176
OB, 176
oblique, 90, 176
obstetrics, 176
obstructive sleep apnea, 176
occipital lobe, 176
Oct., 177
octagon, 175
October, 177
oculus dexter, 177
oculus uterque, 177
OD, 177
ointment, 177
olecranon process, 177
OOB, 178
OOC, 179
oopherectomy, 179
open reduction, internal fixation, 178
operating room, 178
OR, 178
ORIF, 178
OSA, 176
OSHA, 112, 217
osteoporosis, 128, 146
OTC, 179
otoscope, 178
OU, 177
ounce, 179
out of bed, 178

out of control, 179
ovarian, 179
ovaries, 179
over the counter, 179
oximetry, 179
oxygen, 180
oxygen tank, 180
oxygen tubing, 180
oz., 179

P

pacemaker, 182
pacifier, 182
packed red blood cells, 182
PACU, 193
palm, 182
palmistry, 182
palpation, 18
PALS, 186
pancreas, 183
pancreatitis, 183
pants, 183
paper clip, 183
paper towels, 184
parathyroid, 184
parentheses, 184
parietal lobe, 184
partial fill tubing, 185
patella, 145, 185
patellar, 185
patient-controlled analgesia, 185
PBX, 195
PCA, 185
PCN, 187
PCP, 188
PDR, 189
PEA, 197
peanut butter, 186
Pearl Harbor Day, 216
pectoral, 186
Pediatric Advanced Life Support, 186
pee bottle, 254
PEEP, 192
PEG, 187

PEJ, 187
pelvis, 186
pen, 30, 39, 109, 181
pencil, 181
penicillin, 187
percutaneous endoscopic jejunostomy, 187
percutaneous transluminal coronary
    angioplasty, 187
perineum, 187
peripherally inserted central catheter, 187
peritonitis, 23
PERL, 196
per os, 14, 171
personal protective equipment, 188, 212
PET, 192
PFTs, 197
pharyngeal, 188
pharynx, 188
phencyclidine, 188
phosphate, 188
physical therapy, 25, 188
Physician's Desk Reference®, 189
PICC, 187
pig, 189
pill, 189
pill bottle, 189
pillow, 190
pinkeye, 77
pinkie, 190
pituitary hormones, 120
placenta, 190
place setting, 190
plaid, 191
plate, 11, 191
platelets, 191
plts., 191
p.m., 193
pneumocystis, 188
p.o., 188
PO4, 188
POCT, 191
point, 191
point-of-care testing, 191
polka dots, 191
pollex, 192, 238

polycythemia, 206
ponytail, 192
pork, 192
Posey® vest, 259
positive, 193
positive end-expiratory pressure, 14, 192
positron emission tomography, 192
post-anesthesia care unit, 193
post merideum, 193
post-traumatic stress disorder, 193
pot, 193, 264
potassium, 193
potassium chloride, 193
potassium hydroxide, 194
potassium phosphate, 194
potty chair, 42, 75, 194
pound, 194
povidone-iodine, 194
PPD, 198
PPE, 188
PRBCs, 182
premature ventricular contraction, 194
prescription, 195
P-R interval, 195
private branch exchange system, 195
prn, 195
prone, 195
pro re nata, 195
prostatic specific antigen, 195
prosthesis, 196
prosthetic, 196
proximal, 196
PSA, 195
P.T., 188
PTCA, 187
PTSD, 193
pudding, 196
pulmonary function tests, 197
pulmonic valve, 197
pulseless electrical activity, 197
pulse ox, 179, 197
pupils, 197
pupils equal and reactive to light, 196
pureed, 30, 38, 144
purified protein derivative, 198

purse, 198
PVC, 194

Q

Q, 199-200
QD, 201
QHS, 200
QID, 202
QOD, 200
QRS, 200
QS, 201
Q-T, 200
QTc, 201
Q-T interval, 200
Q-tip®, 79
quadriceps, 201
quantity sufficient, 201
quaque die, 201
quart, 202
quater in die, 202
queen, 199
quotation marks, 202

R

rabbit, 203
radial, 204
radiation, 204
radiology, 270
radius, 204
rapid ventricular response, 204
razor, 204-5
razor blade, 205
RBC, 206
RCA, 208
receiving blanket, 205
rectal tube, 205
rectangular, 205
red blood cells, 206
reflex hammer, 206
registered nurse, 206
regulator, 207
renal, 21, 48, 63, 70
respirator, 151, 207, 257

respiratory rate, 207
retina, 207
retinopathy, 207
review of systems, 208
rhabdomyolysis, 80
ribs, 208
right angle, 27, 208
right coronary artery, 208
ring, 209
ring finger, 209
RN, 206
robe, 209
ROS, 208
ROSC, 208
rotator cuff, 209
roughage, 257
RR, 207
RT, 207
rubber band, 210
ruler, 210
RVR, 204
Rx, 195

S

sacral, 212
sacrum, 212
safety goggles, 212
safety pin, 212
salt, 212
sandals, 212
Sat., 213
saturation of peripheral oxygen, 213
Saturday, 213
SB, 220
scalp, 213
scalpel, 205, 213
scapula, 20, 214
scapular, 214
scar, 214
SCDs, 216
SCIP, 229
scissors, 214
scoliosis, 215
scrubs, 215

second, 215
Sept., 215
September, 215
sequential compression devices, 216
sesamoid bone, 185
seventh, 216
sexually transmitted disease, 216
Sharpie®, 109
sharps container, 213, 216
shellfish, 217
shins, 217
shirt, 217
shoes, 217
short of breath, 218
shorts, 218
shoulder blade, 214, 218
shoulders, 218
shrimp, 219
side, 149
siderails, 219
sigmoid colon, 219
sigmoidoscopy, 219
signaling, 61
silverware, 220
sink, 220
sinus bradycardia, 220
sinus rhythm, 56, 220
sinus tachycardia, 220
sixth, 221
skeleton, 221
skin popping, 228
skull, 14, 80, 135, 184, 213, 221
SL, 228
SLE, 230
sling, 221
slippers, 221
smile, 222
smiley face, 126, 222
snake, 222
SOB, 218
socks, 222
sodium, 222
specimen cup, 223
spider, 223
spider bite, 223

spinal, 224
spinal tap, 154, 223
spine, 38, 224
spit pan, 101, 224
spleen, 224
SpO2, 179, 197, 213
spoon, 145, 224, 234
SQ, 228
square, 225
SR, 220
ST, 220
stapler, 225
staples, 225
star, 211
STAT, 33, 225
statim, 225
STD, 216
S-T elevation, 225
sterile towel, 226
sternal, 226
sternum, 53, 226
stethoscope, 226
stomach, 43, 226
stool, 227
straw, 227
stripe, 227
striped, 227
subcutaneous, 228
subendocardial myocardial infarction, 172
suction, 228
suitcase, 228
sulfate, 228
Sunday, 228
supine, 228
suppository, 229
Surgical Care Improvement Project, 229
sutures, 229
swab, 79, 229
sweater, 230
sx, 228
syphilis, 257
syringe, 55, 64, 134, 153, 230
systemic lupus erythrematosus, 230

T

t., 234
T, 232
T4, 236
tablespoon, 232
tablet, 232
tailbone, 73, 232
tampon, 233
tape, 233
tarsal, 233
tarsus, 27, 233
tattoo, 233
TB, 248
tea, 234
teaspoon, 234
teeth, 88, 234
telephone, 235
telephone operator, 195
television, 235
temp, 235
temperature, 235
temporal lobe, 235
tenth, 235
ter in die, 235
testicles, 236
testicular, 236
tetanus, 92
tetraiodothyronine, 236
Thanksgiving, 172, 238
thermometer, 236
thigh, 237
third, 237
30 degrees, 237
thorax, 238
throat, 238
Thu., 238
thumb, 192, 238
Thursday, 172, 238
thymus gland, 239
thyroid, 239
thyroid stimulating hormone, 239
TIA, 245
TIBC, 244
tibia, 239

TID, 235
tissue plasminogen activator, 239
tissues, 240
TMP-SMX, 240
TNTC, 243
toenail, 240
toes, 241
toilet, 241
toilet paper, 241
tongue, 242
tongue blade, 242
tongue depressor, 242
tonsils, 243
too numerous to count, 243
toothbrush, 243
toothpaste, 243
toothpick, 243
on top, 178
torso, 244, 248
total iron-binding capacity, 244
total parenteral nutrition, 244
tourniquet, 244
towel, 245
toxic shock syndrome, 233
tPA, 239
TPN, 244
trachea, 24, 245
tracheal, 245
train, 231
transient ischemic attack, 245
transurethral resection of the prostate, 245
trapezius, 246
trapezoid, 246
trash can, 246
treatment, 246
triangle, 246
triangular, 246
triceps, 247
tricuspid valve, 247
trimethoprim-sulfamethoxazole, 240
tripod, 247
trochanter, 248
truncal, 248
trunk, 244, 248
TSH, 14, 239

tuberculosis, 248
Tues., 248
Tuesday, 248
TV, 235
tweezers, 249
2 × 2, 249
tx, 246

U

ulna, 252
umbilical cord, 252
umbilicus, 43, 252
umbrella, 252
underarm, 253
underneath, 253
underwear, 253
uneven, 150
ung, 177
unguent, 177
unicorn, 251
UO, 254
upper respiratory infection, 254
URI, 254
urinal, 254
urinary tract infection, 254
urine output, 254
urosepsis, 254
USA, 11, 253
uterus, 67, 108, 190, 254
UTI, 254
uvula, 254

V

vacuum cleaner, 256
Valentine's Day, 109
vancomycin-resistant enterococcus, 256
vase, 256
vasoconstriction, 256
vasodilation, 257
vasopressin, 29
VDRL, 257
vegetables, 257
venereal disease, 216, 257

venous thromboembolism, 257
ventilator, 151, 207, 257
ventricle, 258
ventricular, 258
ventricular fibrillation, 258
ventricular tachycardia, 258
vest restaint, 259
vest restraint, 259
VF, 258
vial, 259
violin, 255
vital signs, 259
voice box, 22, 149, 259
VRE, 256
VT, 216, 229, 257-58
VTE, 257

W

waist, 262
walk, 20, 25, 62, 81, 148, 196, 202, 209, 262
walker, 262
wallet, 262
washcloth, 263
watch, 263
water, 261, 263
water breaking, 25
water pitcher, 263
WDL, 265-66
Wed., 263
Wednesday, 263
weed, 193, 264
week, 264
wet floor, 264
wheat cereal, 108, 264
wheelchair, 265
whiplash, 169
wig, 265
window, 265
windpipe, 245, 265
within defined limits, 265
within normal limits, 266
WNL, 265-66
worm, 266
wrench, 266

wrist, 63, 266
wristband, 166, 267
wrist restraints, 267

X

xiphoid process, 270
x-ray, 270
xylophone, 269

Y

Yankauer, 272
yardstick, 271
yogurt, 272

Z

zero, 273
zigzag, 274
zinc, 274

Book description

This is a picture dictionary-style book for anyone interested in the type of English language used in American hospitals. Arranged alphabetically, each of its twenty-six chapters is devoted to one letter of the English alphabet. The content of the images includes abbreviations, anatomy, clothing and personal hygiene, cultural trivia, descriptors, disease, equipment, food, medications, months of the year, numbers, procedures, shapes, and signs. Each item is accompanied by a definition, phonetic spelling, and sample sentence. Images are situated on one half of each page with the texts on the other. An index in the back of the book can be used as a cross-reference tool and to help locate words quickly. Many of the phrases resemble those that may be encountered during classes or examinations for various health-care occupations. It can be useful as a reference tool or exercise book by professionals as well as nonprofessionals. It is designed to be an introduction to hospital work and language for all levels of native and nonnative speakers of English.

Made in the USA
San Bernardino, CA
02 June 2015